A COMMUNITY
HEALTH APPROACH
TO THE ASSESSMENT
OF INFANTS AND
THEIR PARENTS

A COMMUNITY HEALTH APPROACH TO THE ASSESSMENT OF INFANTS AND THEIR PARENTS

The CARE Programme

Kevin Browne
Jo Douglas
Catherine Hamilton-Giachritsis
Jean Hegarty

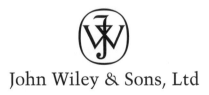

John Wiley & Sons, Ltd

Other Wiley Editorial Offices

John Wiley & Sons Inc., 111 River Street, Hoboken, NJ 07030, USA
Jossey-Bass, 989 Market Street, San Francisco, CA 94103-1741, USA
Wiley-VCH Verlag GmbH, Boschstr. 12, D-69469 Weinheim, Germany
John Wiley & Sons Australia Ltd, 42 McDougall Street, Milton, Queensland 4064, Australia
John Wiley & Sons (Asia) Pte Ltd, 2 Clementi Loop #02-01, Jin Xing Distripark, Singapore
129809
John Wiley & Sons Canada Ltd, 22 Worcester Road, Etobicoke, Ontario, Canada M9W 1L1

Wiley also publishes its books in a variety of electronic formats. Some content that appears
in print may not be available in electronic books.

Library of Congress Cataloging-in-Publication Data

A community health approach to the assessment of infants and their parents: the care
programme / Kevin Browne . . . [et al.].
        p.   cm.
    Includes bibliographical references and index.
    ISBN-13: 978-0-470-09251-4 (cloth: alk. paper)
    ISBN-10: 0-470-09251-3 (cloth: alk. paper)
    ISBN-13: 978-0-470-09252-1 (pbk.: alk. paper)
    ISBN-10: 0-470-09252-1 (pbk.: alk. paper)
    1. Community mental health services.   2. Infant health services.   3. Maternal health
services.   4. Child development.   I. Browne, Kevin.
    RA790.5.C662 2006
    362.198′92–dc22   2006011226

British Library Cataloguing in Publication Data

A catalogue record for this book is available from the British Library

ISBN-13   978-0-470-09251-4 (hbk) 978-0-470-09252-1 (pbk)
ISBN-10   0-470-09251-3 (hbk) 0-470-09252-1 (pbk)

Typeset in 10/12pt Palatino by SNP Best-set Typesetter Ltd., Hong Kong
Printed and bound in Great Britain by TJ International Ltd, Padstow, Cornwall
This book is printed on acid-free paper responsibly manufactured from sustainable forestry
in which at least two trees are planted for each one used for paper production.

CONTENTS

ABOUT THE AUTHORS

Professor Kevin Browne is a Chartered Psychologist and a Chartered Biologist and is employed by the School of Psychology, at the University of Birmingham, as Director of the Centre for Forensic and Family Psychology. He has been researching family violence and child maltreatment for over 25 years and has published extensively on these subjects, acting as co-editor (with Margaret Lynch) of *Child Abuse Review* from 1992 to 1999. His most recent co-edited book is *Early Prediction and Prevention of Child Abuse: A Handbook* (Wiley, 2002). After 12 years as an Executive Councillor of the International Society for the Prevention of Child Abuse and Neglect (ISPCAN), he is currently Consultant to the European Commission, World Bank and the WHO on child protection strategies and to the WHO and UNICEF on training in the public health approach to the prevention of child abuse and neglect. He has worked and presented in over 47 countries worldwide, having spent two and a half years as Chief Executive of the High Level Group for Romanian Children. In support of international work, his book entitled *Preventing Family Violence* (co-authored with Martin Herbert, Wiley, 1997) has been translated into Chinese, Japanese and Polish and his papers on the topic into Greek, Turkish, Romanian, Russian, Slovak, French, Italian and Spanish. His current research interests are the influence of media violence on children and teenagers, the concept of victim to offender and the effects of early institutional care on child development and adult behaviour.

Jo Douglas is a Consultant Clinical Psychologist who has specialised in working with children and families over the past 30 years. She was Head of the Psychology Service at Great Ormond Street Hospital in London and Honorary Senior Lecturer at the Institute of Child Health (University of London). She has worked extensively with a wide range of childhood emotional and behavioural problems and has written books and articles for both parents and professionals. She is well known for her work with managing sleeping and eating problems in young children and has lectured and trained primary and secondary health care staff across the country in these skills. She is now an independent psychologist.

Dr Catherine Hamilton-Giachritsis is a Chartered Forensic Psychologist and Senior Lecturer in Forensic Psychology at the University of Birmingham. Previously she worked in Birmingham Social Services Psychology Department, undertaking assessments of families where there was considered to be a risk to children, or assessing the needs of children and adolescents in such families. She is co-author of the Wiley volume 'Early Prediction and Prevention of Child Abuse: A Handbook' (2002). In addition, Catherine has published widely on child maltreatment, family violence, the institutionalisation of infants and young children, and the links between media violence and crime. Catherine is chair of the West Midlands branch of the British Association for the Study and Prevention of Child Abuse and Neglect (BASPCAN West Midlands) and is currently engaged in further training in clinical psychology.

Jean Hegarty has had a long career working with children and their families. Her experience has encompassed midwifery practice and nursing sick children. For the past 23 years, Jean has worked in the community specialising in preventative approaches to health care for children and their families. She practiced as a Health visitor prior to becoming the Designated nurse for Child protection in Southend-on-Sea from 1988–1998. Jean's last appointment prior to leaving the N.H.S was as a Sure Start programme manager in Southend. During Jean's time in the South East of Essex she successfully worked with her Health visiting colleagues providing training and support. Jean has shared this practice with colleagues throughout the country over the past 13 years. She has spoken at National Nursing conferences and Child protection forums including the International congress on child protection. She currently undertakes Supervision and Consultancy work as an Independent practitioner. Jean would like to convey her high regard for the Health visitors in Southend who worked with her during the development of the programme. This regard is extended to the Social workers, Midwives and Essex Police who were also superb in 'working together' to achieve best practice. Jean remains aware that the fieldwork practitioners gave their commitment to the development of quality services. It is to the practitioners then, that Jean conveys her highest regard for their achievements and for the constant support, gratitude and interest they gave her.

PREFACE

Following the Kennedy (2001) and Laming (2003) reports, which were critical of services for child health in England, the National Service Framework for Children, Young People and Maternity Services (Dept of Health, 2004) outlines a ten year programme to improve services for children and their families. The national standards set within the framework advocate a fundamental change in the design and delivery of children's services across health, social care and education. 'Services are child-centred and look at the whole child – not just the illness or the problem' (Dept of Health, 2004, p. 2). The NSF for children also emphasises the needs of vulnerable children in society and refers to high profile cases of fatal child abuse (e.g., Laming, 2003). Consequently, it advocates early assessment and intervention that are both comprehensive and timely, to improve access to services for children and families according to their needs.

The book describes, in detail, a method of assessment and intervention for young children and their families entitled the Child Assessment Rating and Evaluation (CARE) programme. Characteristics of the infant, the parents, the family and the environment in which they live are used to identify need and guide further interventions by a variety of professionals. The focus of the model is the early prediction and prevention of problems for child health, development and protection. The emphasis is upon the principle of partnership with parents.

The CARE programme developed as a pragmatic attempt to deal with limited resources in community services and how best to apply those limited resources to maximum effect. Consequently, a 'risk approach' emerged, where all families are briefly assessed by community nurses visiting the home (midwives and health visitors), who identify those families in need of further support and help. These families are recognised as those of highest priority for services to meet the needs of the child and ameliorate any family difficulties in meeting those needs.

The model is best applied within a universal community service offered by trained health/social service professionals, such as midwives and health visitors, as a part of their normal primary care services and incurring no further costs. Using a universal service of home visits to families with new-borns as a foundation, families with factors associated with increased 'need' can be recognised. Targeted services can then be offered in addition to the standard, universal service already received by all families. On occasion, the need of the child and their family will be so urgent and/or extensive that specialist services will be required. These specialist services aim to respond to any current or underlying situation that has the potential to significantly harm the child. Specialist services are offered in conjunction with targeted and universal services already received.

The majority of the work on methods for 'targeting' families with maximum sensitivity and specificity was carried out by staff at the Centre for Forensic and Family Psychology, University of Birmingham. However, this book represents the culmination of more than a decade of work developing a health practice-based approach to assessing the needs of children and their families in the community, and intervening in the community to support and prevent undesirable outcomes for children. It owes a lot to the imagination and foresight of Jean Hegarty, who placed this work within health visiting practices. Under her supervision, many of the ideas derived from academic research have been successfully translated into practice in Essex (1995–2005), mainly within the Southend-on-Sea health care setting and the Sure Start programme.

The aim of this book is to make these ideas available to a wider audience in order to inform policy and practice. We also felt it was important to demonstrate the research and thought behind the model so that professionals can have an understanding of how the programme was developed based on evidence. For grammatical simplicity, we have referred to midwives and health visitors as female throughout the book, reflecting the fact that the majority of health professionals are female. However, we readily acknowledge that the community nurse's role does not relate to gender and the reader should equally apply our comments to both male and female community nurses.

Kevin Browne, Jo Douglas, Catherine Hamilton-Giachritsis
and Jean Hegarty
January 2005

The forms and booklets in Appendices 1–5 are also available online, free to purchasers of the book. Visit www.wiley.com/go/care to access and download these materials.

ACKNOWLEDGEMENTS

In 2003, Jean Hegarty (nee Ware), the Programme Manager for Sure Start in Southend invited Jo Douglas to look at the work she had been involved with as a health visitor and a designated nurse for child protection over many years. Jo initially became involved with the CARE programme in her role as Consultant Child Clinical Psychologist. Jean was keen and had the strategic foresight to recognise how incredibly important the Child Assessment Rating and Evaluation programme (CARE; Browne, Hamilton & Ware, 1995) is and wanted a book written in order to disseminate the ideas that had developed in the CARE approach to community nursing and primary care and to promote good practice.

Jean was the instigator and had the drive to conceive this book and Jo was invited to write it in collaboration with Kevin Browne and Catherine Hamilton-Giachritsis. Kevin, Catherine and Jean had developed and researched methods of assessing risk factors for child protection referrals in infants and their families in Essex using risk factors in combination with observations of parenting and indicators of attachment. This was a significant advance on the purely risk factor approach that was first developed by Kevin in the Surrey area (Browne & Saqi, 1988a).

It was agreed that all four of us would pool our resources to create a book that would provide useful clinical, evidence-based practice guidelines for community nurses. However, we are indebted to Jean for the confidence and support she has shown throughout the ten years of CARE development and implementation. We are also indebted to Jo for kick-starting the process of writing this book by pulling together all the materials that had been developed over ten years into a coherent structure.

In addition, we must mention Carol Steff, Senior Health Visitor and Team Leader for Sure Start in Southend, for her invaluable help in discussing cases and supporting us in understanding the impact of the programme on the clinical practice in Essex. Also, thanks to Terry Fultan, midwife, who has used this programme very successfully in her practice and has shared some of her findings about the process. Jo has also received invaluable clinical information from the team of health visitors and Sure Start workers at

Southend during their fascinating and illuminating supervision sessions. Jo is extremely grateful and feels privileged to have been able to join with them in thinking about many of the tremendously difficult and distressing clinical issues they have to cope with on a daily basis.

The book has now finally arrived after a long gestation. We only hope that this new arrival will continue to flourish and influence clinical practice in the forthcoming years and go forth and multiply!

Kevin Browne, Jo Douglas, Catherine Hamilton-Giachritsis and Jean Hegarty

1

INTRODUCTION: CHILDCARE AND PROTECTION – A PUBLIC HEALTH APPROACH

Most countries offer at least some services to children and their families, especially around the time of birth. In those countries with more developed health care systems, this usually includes community support and home visits by health professionals. These health professionals are at the front-line in promoting the rights of children as they enter the world. Following the United Nations Convention on the Rights of the Child (UNCRC, 1989), one of the most important aspects of community support is helping the parent(s) to recognise the importance of registering the child as a legal entity in the local community and, indeed, the national population. A child's identity (usually secured by a certificate of registration at birth) opens the opportunity to health and education provision, at the same time as protecting the child against abduction and trafficking.

Having established a child's identity, the right to survival and development is further enhanced by the child and family's registration with primary health care services, usually through a general practitioner or family doctor. The child's right to health care up to the age of 18 years is then usually secured, although in some countries this is means tested with free services only available to children of parents on low income.

Health and social services for parents are also associated with the rights of the child, as the UNCRC (1989) clearly states that the child has the right to grow up in his or her own biological family. In addition, services should be made available to families in order to ensure their capacity to meet the child's social, emotional and developmental needs (Article 19, UNCRC, 1989). Only as a last resort when, despite services offered, parents fail to meet their child's needs and the child is at risk of significant harm, is it recommended that the child should be removed from the family and placed in alternative family care (on a temporary or permanent basis). Adoption is only recommended when it is in the long-term best interests of the child.

In the UK, the Children Act (1989, 2004) closely follows the principles of the UNCRC (1989) and many of the above rights and services offered are taken for granted by the population because free health and social care is available. The government has highlighted the role of professional responsibility and inter-agency communication when 'Working to Safeguard Children' (Dept of Health, Home Office, Dept for Education and Employment, 1999). This concept has recently been emphasised and reinforced in the publication 'Keeping Children Safe' (Dept of Health et al., 2003), which represents the government's response to the inquiry into the death of Victoria Climbié due to horrendous abuse and neglect (Laming, 2003). This inquiry had a major impact on the recent 'Every Child Matters' initiative (Dept for Education and Skills, 2004a).

It remains the Local Authority's responsibility to safeguard and promote the welfare of children who are 'in need' and to support parents to care for their children within a family environment. Therefore, health professionals should work closely with the Local Authority and social services to provide a range of interventions related to family crisis and support, positive parenting skills, prevention of child abuse and neglect, and promoting optimal development in children with physical and intellectual disabilities.

The current focus for child care and protection is early prediction and prevention, as well as timely interventions through preventative services. This can most appropriately be achieved by considering child care and protection in the wider context of child welfare. Each local community is planned to have child and family centres and closer involvement with schools to address the needs of children and their families. However, there is still an emphasis in the UK on social care and education being the key agencies for child care and protection. The public health approach has been neglected, with the role of health professionals limited to inter-agency collaboration on health and medical issues. This chapter advocates refocusing the debate, putting the health sector first as the key agency in the early prediction and prevention of child adversity. Indeed, health professionals are the front line in promoting children's optimal health and development.

THE PUBLIC HEALTH APPROACH

The World Health Organisation (1998a, 1999) defines a public health approach as the viewing of child abuse and neglect within the broader context of child welfare, families and communities. From a Health Service perspective, this requires the integration of good practices within three areas of service provision to families and children: safe pregnancy and childbirth, the management of childhood health and illness, and targeting services for families who have a high number of risk factors associated with child abuse and neglect.

Safe Pregnancy and Childbirth

The following guidelines are adapted from the World Health Organisation (1998b) as ways of providing services to ensure safe pregnancy and childbirth:

- Pre-birth: prenatal screening of the foetus for abnormalities (using ultrasound) and the promotion of healthy life-styles in the mother in order to protect the foetus (e.g., reducing maternal substance misuse, managing physical and mental illness) should be undertaken.
- During birth: natural delivery and the use of appropriate technology should be promoted, as should encouraging significant others (usually the father) to be present to support the mother and skin contact between mother and baby immediately following birth. The aim is to promote positive birth experiences for parents, which in turn encourage parental bonding to the infant.
- After birth: 24-hour access of significant others to the mother and child in the maternity unit, appropriate neonatal care and advice on practical parenting skills (e.g., breast feeding, bathing, etc.) should be standard because promotion of sensitive parenting can occur through positive post-birth experiences.

Midwifery nurses are best placed to provide continuity of care to pregnant mothers. This involves the same midwife offering individualised support with pre-birth home visits, assistance in childbirth and infant care throughout pregnancy until 10 days after birth. This is regarded as the 'best practice' model for promoting natural childbirth and parental bonding. In terms of child protection, such an approach increases the likelihood of positive parenting and thereby limits the possibility of infant abandonment, poor parenting, insecure attachment and child maltreatment.

Integrated Management of Childhood Health and Illness

The management of child health and illness by primary health care teams and community health nurses is aimed at the prevention of child disability, morbidity and mortality, as well as at limiting the stress to parents in caring for a sick child. However, children coming to the attention of health services through home or clinic visits also offer the potential to screen for the possibility of maltreatment.

All children having contact with the health service can be observed and checked in the normal way for physical injuries and illnesses. However, during the examination, the possibility of non-accidental injury and illnesses occurring because of abuse and/or neglect should be kept in mind. In the absence of a standardised screening tool, history taking by doctors and nurses on the condition of the child should include the following components to promote identification of and protection from child abuse and neglect:

- history of family circumstances (e.g., presence of isolation, violence, addiction or mental illness)
- history of child's condition (e.g., story doesn't explain injury, delay in seeking help)
- child's physical condition when undressed (e.g., presence of disability, lesions or genital discharge)
- child's physical care (e.g., cleanliness, teeth, hair, nails, hygiene)
- child's behaviour (e.g., frozen hyper-vigilance or aggressive hyperactivity)
- parent's/caretaker's behaviour and demeanour (e.g., low self-esteem, depressed, over anxious, insensitive, careless, punishing, defensive).

Child Care and Protection

It is suggested that child protection services should focus on preventative and protective strategies, offering interventions to families with a high number of risk factors associated with child abuse and neglect. If possible, the services should be targeted to these families before maltreatment begins. According to the Department of Health et al. (2000), health and social care services should assess families in the following holistic way:

- assessment of children's development needs in general
- assessment of the capacity of the parent(s) to respond appropriately to their child's needs
- assessment of the wider social and environmental factors that impact on the capacity to parent.

This is known as the 'Lilac Book' assessment format. Risk factors are identified from 'undesirable' characteristics associated with the child, the parents and the family environment.

RECENT DEVELOPMENTS

Following the public health approach advocated by the World Health Organ-isation (*Health in the 21st Century*, WHO, 2000), recent government guidelines (Dept of Health, 2004) have adopted a similar perspective in their 10-year plan for integrated services offered to children and their families. The national standards outlined are applied to the following topics:

1. Promoting health and well-being, identifying needs and intervening early.
2. Supporting parenting.
3. Child, young person and family-centred services.
4. Growing up into adulthood.
5. Safeguarding and promoting the welfare of children and young people.
6. Children and young people who are ill.
7. Children and young people in hospital.
8. Disabled children and young people and those with complex health needs.
9. The mental health and psychological well-being of children and young people.
10. Medicines for children and young people.
11. Maternity services.

The implementation of the National Service Framework for Children is part of a broader commitment (*'Every Child Matters'*) to promote a programme of 'Change for Children', improving standards of care and support that will enhance optimal outcomes for children and their families (Dept for Educa-tion and Skills & Dept of Health, 2004; Dept for Education and Skills, 2004b). This commitment promises to support all children to achieve the following outcomes:

- be healthy
- stay safe
- enjoy and achieve
- make a positive contribution
- achieve economic well-being.

The best way to promote these outcomes is to prevent problems from begin-ning through effective intervention and support for children and their fami-lies. This gives children the best possible chance to realise their optimal potential and ensure they make a positive contribution to society and achieve a happy life with economic well-being as they grow older. In addition, the

NSF for Children acknowledges that such children will grow up to be better equipped for parenting their own children. The Every Child Matters initiative (DfES, 2004c, d) further recognises the well-established premise that positive parenting and early intervention may contribute to reducing the number of children who engage in delinquency and crime as teenagers (Browne & Herbert, 1997; Patterson, DeBaryshe & Ramsey, 1989). The topic of child protection exemplifies the way early interventions can promote the health and safety of children, and set them on the right developmental path.

ADVANTAGES OF EARLY INTERVENTION

The importance of early intervention can be considered from two, very different perspectives: the impact on children and the financial cost to society.

In the UK, it is generally agreed that at least two children per week die as a result of child maltreatment, with a further two suffering permanent disability, with infants most at risk of fatal injury (Browne & Lynch, 1995; Reder & Duncan, 2002). However, younger children are particularly vulnerable to abuse and/or neglect. Indeed, in 2003 the highest rate of registration on the Child Protection Register in England and Wales was for physical abuse and neglect in young children under one year (51 per 10,000; Dept of Health, 2004b). Therefore, it is essential that prediction and prevention occur from birth.

The financial costs of child abuse and neglect include both costs for the short- and long-term treatment of victims and the less apparent impact on other areas of society. The World Health Organisation (1999) highlighted a number of areas for inclusion in calculations of cost. These were medical care for victims, mental health provision for victims, legal costs for public childcare, criminal justice and prosecution costs, treatment of offenders, Social Work provision and specialist education. Overall, it has been estimated that the total economic cost in the United Kingdom is £735 million per annum (National Commission for the Prevention of Child Abuse, 1996), compared to $12,410 million per annum in the USA (WHO, 1999). These costs may have increased over the past ten years, since both estimates relate to 1996 figures.

The incredible cost of child protection once child abuse and neglect has occurred justifies more expenditure on preventative measures and services to support children and their families.

PREVENTION OF CHILD ABUSE AND NEGLECT

Strategies for the prevention of child maltreatment fall into three categories: primary (aimed at the whole population), secondary (targeting groups) and tertiary (after maltreatment has occurred).

Primary Prevention

Primary prevention is aimed at the whole population. Teachers, General Practitioners, practice nurses, health visitors and nursery workers are all important in providing appropriate advice and support. For example, community nurses (health visitors) have on-going contact with all children less than five years old in terms of providing advice on practical parenting skills, health and parental well-being.

Primary prevention services offered to everyone within the population include home visits by health workers, education of parents and care-givers, school programmes on parenting and child development, day nursery places, telephone help-lines and drop-in community centres. The purpose of this support is to assist positive parenting skills and to encourage the development of a secure attachment between parent and child. Secure attachments are highly significant in the early prevention of child maltreatment, first, because of the long-term positive impact on child development it engenders (e.g., positive self-image). Second, in situations where a high number of risk factors for child maltreatment are present, child abuse and neglect are more likely to occur in the absence of secure, positive attachments (Morton & Browne, 1998).

Many initiatives aimed at promoting positive parenting now exist (Sure Start in England; Triple P in Australia, Sanders & Cann, 2002). However, other strategies can be used regularly by primary health professionals, even in the absence of a full programme. Indeed, promoting positive parenting skills and sensitivity can be achieved in a straightforward manner, for example, just by raising awareness of verbal abuse and the implications of this on the development of a positive self-image in the child (see Table 1.1).

From a public health perspective, prevention begins with professional awareness of issues such as the mental health needs of the parent(s), negative aspects of peri-natal care and the importance of secure attachments. In turn, primary care professionals can utilise this information in their work

Table 1.1 Primary prevention by promoting positive parenting

Harsh words hurt	Kind words help
• SHUT UP	• PLEASE
• STOP IT	• WELL DONE
• GO AWAY	• YOU'RE CLEVER
• YOU'RE STUPID	• YOU'RE GOOD
• YOU'RE BAD	• I LOVE YOU
• WISH YOU WERE NEVER BORN	

with parents and pass on appropriate knowledge to those parents. For example, providing information to parents on how to cope with post-natal depression; the dangers of shaking or roughly handling a newborn; and educating parents about the development of attachment processes.

The development of secure attachments, being complex, will be considered in more detail. The importance of imparting knowledge of this process to parents is to assist them in understanding the needs of their child and temperamental differences. For the purposes of parental understanding, this can be separated into three stages:

- Birth: parent to infant bonding is a result of the psychological availability of the parent and the genetic pre-dispositions of the child to respond to the parent. This may occur immediately after birth or take some time to develop within the first six months (see Sluckin, Herbert & Sluckin, 1983).
- 5–12 months: formulation of infant to parent bond (infant attachment) with maturity where the child shows a preference for the primary care-giver, demonstrates some distress when left by the primary care-giver and is comforted by the presence of the primary care-giver. The infant uses the primary care-giver as a base for exploration and as a source of imitation (see Bowlby, 1969).
- 12–24 months: infant attachment quality (secure/insecure) is measurable and observable, and can be classified into a) insecure and avoidant, b1) secure and independent, b2) secure and dependent, c) insecure and ambivalent, d) disorganised (see Morton & Browne, 1998).

It is important, however, for professionals to remain aware that, whilst providing simple explanations to parents might assist in development of attachment, the assessment of attachment is not simplistic and requires appropriate training. A common misperception is to refer to a child as 'attached'. Nearly all children are attached in some form, it is the quality of infant attachment which is of interest, i.e., secure or insecure. Maccoby (1980) describes how the quality of attachment in a child is dependent on the levels of acceptance, accessibility, consistency, sensitivity and co-operation of the primary care-giver (usually the natural mother). Whilst at times this can appear to be 'common-sense', it does not *always* follow that a maltreated child is insecurely attached to their primary care-giver, or that a child who clings to their mother is securely attached. However, it is more common for maltreated, abused and neglected children to be less securely attached and usually to show patterns of insecurity and stranger anxiety. Indeed, a meta-analysis of 13 studies showed insecure attachment to the mother in 76% of maltreated samples compared to 34% of non-maltreated samples (Morton & Browne, 1998). The long-term consequences of insecure attachments in early childhood have now been clearly recognised and described. They may be summarised as follows (Cassidy & Shaver, 1999; Simpson & Rholes, 1998; Solomon & George, 1999):

- The early carer-infant relationship is internalised by the child and may be the 'prototype' or 'model' to which all future relationships are assimilated and are based upon.
- The child is likely to develop an image of him/herself as unworthy of love and affection and lacking control over his/her environment.
- Maltreated, abused and neglected children may have greater problems forming relationships with siblings, peers, intimate partners and their own children in future.

It is important to recognise that the transition to parenthood is a critical period in adult psychological development. Support should be provided to parents who are unable to cope, by primary care teams who may refer to telephone help lines, drop-in centres, community support groups and voluntary groups, as well as specialist health and social services. Hence, multidisciplinary training is required to enable primary care professionals to recognise and intervene with parental low self-esteem, anxiety, depression and alcohol/drug misuse. All these factors strongly influence the quality of parental care and infant attachment. This, in turn, increases the risk of child maltreatment and development in the child of poor internal models of relationships and feelings of low self-worth.

Secondary Prevention

Secondary prevention involves targeting resources to families identified as being 'high priority' for additional services. The aim of the 'risk approach' of proactive surveillance is to identify children at risk and offer health services and referral to social services before maltreatment occurs. Such an approach has the potential to prevent victimisation from ever beginning. Again, primary care professionals and teachers provide the first point of contact with the child and can be alert to signs of potential child maltreatment. For example, doctors and/or community nurses make home visits to monitor child health. At the same time, they have the opportunity to screen for socio-demographic and psychological risk factors for child abuse and neglect.

When the number and severity of risk factors present pass a threshold, child protection services are offered automatically. However, it is important not to stigmatise families who have yet to harm their child(ren) and targeting these families should be based on the principle of priority for services.

Therefore, families should be considered as 'high priority' or 'low priority' for social service referral and/or health service input (e.g., substance misuse programmes or mental health care), rather than regarded as 'high risk' or 'low risk' for child abuse and neglect.

Browne and Herbert (1997) describe additional assessments that go beyond a simple risk factor checklist to be more 'sensitive' to families with the potential for child abuse and neglect (hits) from those who have a high number of risk factors in combination with protection factors that reduce their chances of child maltreatment (false positives). This is based upon an evaluation of the parent-child relationship. These included:

- caretaker's knowledge and attitudes to parenting the child
- parental perceptions of the child's behaviour and the child's perception of the parent
- parental emotions and responses to stress
- style of parent-child interaction and behaviour
- quality of child to parent attachment
- quality of parenting.

Tertiary Prevention/Intervention Strategies

Tertiary prevention is the offering of services to children and families where abuse and/or neglect have already occurred. On 31 March 2004, 24 in 10,000 children under 18 years were on child protection registers for actual or likely child abuse and/or neglect in England and Wales (Dept for Education and Skills, 2005). Of these, 41% were registered for neglect, 19% for physical abuse, 9% for sexual abuse, 18% for emotional abuse and 14% for cases of mixed abuse and/or neglect. Overall, 68% of the children on registers were 10 years or younger, with a similar number of boys and girls registered. However, girls suffered more sexual abuse (11%) compared to boys (8%), while boys suffered more physical abuse (16%) than girls (15%). Following the child protection conference, 13% of the children were taken into public care; of these, 79% were placed with foster carers (mainly younger children), 5% were in children's homes or a secure unit (mainly older children), 13% were placed with parents and 3% in other types of placements (Dept for Education and Skills, 2005).

Therefore, reactive surveillance and identification of abused and neglected children leads to intervention both to stop the current maltreatment and to prevent recurrent victimisation. However, intervention at this late stage is not always successful. It has been shown that one in four children referred to police child protection units is re-referred within 27 months for a new incident of child maltreatment (either by the same perpetrator or a different perpetrator), with the rate of re-referral doubling following the second referral (Hamilton & Browne, 1999).

Tertiary prevention is an essential service even in the presence of proactive primary and secondary preventative measures. Although this book emphasises the role of doctors and nurses in the prevention of child abuse and neglect, it is also recognised that they must receive adequate training in the detection and identification of cases when maltreatment has already occurred.

Doctors and nurses when presented with a condition that may be associated with child abuse and neglect (e.g., evidence of physical injury, unusual genital discharge, low birth weight and/or malnutrition, developmental delay or disability) should observe and make notes of any suspicious condition or injury. It is essential to ask for an explanation from the parents for the condition or injury, as well as for any delay in seeking treatment and to judge whether this explanation is consistent or inconsistent with the medical evidence. In the presence of a suspicious physical condition or injury, a delay in seeking help or a lack of consistency with the explanation should generate serious concern and an appropriate urgent referral to specialist child protection services.

Where there is evidence of inadequate physical care of the child or a number of risk factors present associated with the child, the parent or the family, such circumstances would warrant further observation and follow-up similar to a secondary prevention approach. Any abnormal behaviour shown by the child (e.g., frozen watchfulness) or by the parent (e.g., angry and defensive) should also be seen as an indicator that not all may be well in the family, requiring further observation and follow-up home visits.

CONCLUSION

As well as facilitating the development of the child through consistent and sensitive parenting, the parent acts as the child's protection from adversity. Thus, doctors and nurses visiting the family homes need to address their observations to the health and welfare of the parent, as well as the health and welfare of the child. Parental depression and other mental health difficulties reduce the capacity of the parent to care and may seriously limit the optimal development of the child. In addition, alcohol and drug abuse may result in both the physical and emotional neglect of the child(ren). The stress of a violent relationship between parents may also have physical and/or mental health consequences. Hence, primary health care teams and community nurses need to be concerned with family health in order to promote the welfare, development and rights of the child.

OVERVIEW OF THE CARE PROGRAMME – THE FIRST YEAR OF LIFE

The first year of life of a new infant can be a stressful period for many parents as they struggle to find their new identity as parents and get to know their new baby. Their hopes and aspirations for the infant can reflect their own failures and lost dreams or be a springboard of optimism for the future. The birth may be greeted with delight and pride or with worry and regret. A single mother may be angry and resentful that she will have to cope on her own or a couple may hope that the new baby will bind their volatile relationship into a firmer bond. Parents of already large families may wonder how they are going to manage with yet another mouth to feed, whilst the desperate hope for a boy may be shattered with the birth of a girl or there may be fear that the baby will look like the natural father and not the husband. There may also be the desperation felt when disabilities are diagnosed and parents face the loss of a 'normal' baby. Birth is not always a happy time. New parents may not have the support around them from family and friends to help and offer advice. Sadly, isolation, fear and uncertainty may be the paramount feelings of early parenthood making many parents feel they have 'failed'.

During the first year, the baby is vulnerable but demanding. Babies need protection, comfort, feeding, caring, love and undivided attention. They cry when they need something and force their parents into responding without being able to tell them what the problem is. Parents are faced with complex decision making and trying to understand an angry or distressed baby who is screaming in their ear and will not calm down. The stress generated by a young baby can crumble fragile defences, exacerbate feelings of inadequacy or lack of confidence and reinforce a sense of being an inadequate or poor parent. It can also create blame and anger between parents in sharing or managing the baby's demands, highlight how the parents are unable to effectively negotiate with each other and may even make the parents want to run away and hide from the challenge. The parents' loss of independence and the immediate sense of responsibility that the baby generates in them can be frightening. Young parents may experience a rude awakening and may wish to retreat to their previous self-focused world. Fathers may abandon mothers and babies, as they cannot stand the strain and sense of confinement.

Overall, the first year of life is a critical time in coming to terms with being a parent and the changes in your relationship, exacerbated by possible financial problems, issues of returning to work and decisions about childcare arrangements.

A DANGEROUS TIME

The first year of life is also a dangerous time for some babies. Mortality rates are highest around and just after birth; in England and Wales nearly 3,500 infants die each year before they are one year old. The homicide rate for children under one is almost five times greater than the average (Home Office, 2003) and over half of the children that die as a result of child abuse each year do so as a baby (Harker & Kendall, 2003).

Although heightened risk continues into the second year (Durfee & Tilton-Durfee, 1995; Reder & Duncan, 2002), the majority of deaths through abuse are in the first year of life with the perinatal period being particularly important. Risk is high for:

* Babies who are unwanted (Murphy et al., 1985; Oliver, 1983). Important clues in the perinatal period include mothers who consider a termination of the pregnancy; who fail to present for antenatal care; who want the baby to be adopted but change their mind at the last moment; or who carry a baby conceived as the result of incestuous abuse.
* Babies who are born in secret (Bonnet, 1993; Marks & Kumar, 1993). These mothers may not acknowledge that they are pregnant and fail to present for any antenatal care and the baby is either abandoned to die or actively killed.

Sadly, many of these mothers will have been in contact with obstetric, postnatal or community health services prior to the abuse of their infant, but their distress and desperation may not have been noticed, acknowledged or acted upon (Greenland, 1987). Therefore, the role of the community health worker is vitally important in helping identify parents who are having problems adapting to or coping with parenthood. Prevention strategies at the primary health care level could provide effective and timely support at times when parents most need it. An effective assessment strategy is at the basis of any preventative approach so that resources can be targeted to families in need.

EQUALITY OF OPPORTUNITY

Children, sadly, are not born equal. The economic circumstances into which they are born, their health, their intellectual ability, their personality traits and parental expectations of each newborn immediately create differences. Disadvantage can start before birth and is compounded by the significant impact of the parent-child relationship on the infant's development (Harker & Kendall, 2003). However, if the foundation of our society is based on the belief that all individuals are inherently of equal worth then we must strive to create circumstances where all individuals begin life with the same chances. Our commitment to an equal start for all children means that we need to address the unjust inequalities. From the early months of life, the pattern of interaction between a parent and child is heavily influenced by the parent's own wellbeing. This has a lasting impact on the baby's social and emotional development. The Institute for Public Policy Research (Harker & Kendall, 2003) has looked at a wide range of public policy interventions including financial, health and parenting support and has tried to assess the appropriate balance between them in order to consider how public policy should change in order to achieve a more equal start for children. Their view is that in terms of achieving greater equality, no period of life matters more than pregnancy and the first 12 months of life.

Early life experiences strongly influence the way that the brain develops. For example:

- The amount of verbal interaction that parents have with their babies can influence language development and reading ability later in childhood (Balbernie, 2001; Glaser, 2000; Hart & Risley, 1995).
- Differences in cognitive ability are detectable between social classes by the age of 22 months (Feinstein, 1998).
- Experiences of abuse and neglect have been shown to have neurological effects on the developing brain (Glaser, 2000; Schore, 2001a, b).

In addition, the parent-infant interaction is crucial in shaping the child's social and emotional development (Glaser, 2000; Schaffer, 1990). The quality of this interaction is particularly important as it enhances the infant's feelings of self-worth, self-esteem, a sense of belonging and a degree of self-control that can help protect them from the stress of social disadvantage.

All of these issues lead us to recognise the vital importance of influences during pregnancy and the first year of life in the future life of children. Community support services therefore need careful targeting to 'at risk' populations that require support and help to offset the disadvantages that create inequalities.

THE EFFECTS OF PARENTING

Psychological research has not yet been able to produce a unifying theory of parenting but it has been able to produce a range of theories that address particular kinds of parenting and child outcomes (O'Connor, 2002). Some theories examine the parent-child relationship while others focus more on the features of the child and parents as individuals. The dimensions of the parent-child relationships that have most consistently been associated with differences in children's wellbeing include warmth/support or sensitivity/responsiveness, conflict or hostility/rejection and the method and degree of controlling the child's behaviour, i.e. coercive or inductive (Ainsworth et al., 1978; Morton & Browne, 1998; Patterson, 1982).

Attempts to understand why some parents have greater problems than others parenting effectively have focused on developmental and life course risks of the parents, as well as current social and interpersonal stresses (Belsky, 1984; Browne & Herbert, 1997). Although animal studies support the connection between the effects of severe care-giving deprivation and abuse on the subsequent parenting behaviour in the offspring, this has been much harder to study in humans. There is data to indicate that parents who received early institutional care in their childhood have high rates of parenting difficulty (Dept of Health & Quinton, 2004; Quinton et al., 1984; Quinton, 1999). The concept of the inter-generational continuity of parenting disturbance has raised a number of concerns as has the concept of the 'cycle of deprivation', but there is evidence that indicates early childhood experience does influence the parenting capabilities of the adult (Dixon, Browne & Hamilton-Giachritsis, 2005; Dixon, Hamilton-Giachritsis & Browne, 2005).

A new area of research in genetics has queried whether there are genetic influences on individual differences in parenting behaviour, but no clear data in this area yet exists (O'Connor, 2002).

EARLY PARENTING SKILLS

The care of the infant involves a high level of physical care like feeding, changing, clothing and ensuring their physical survival. However, attention to their social and emotional development is equally important. Emde (1989) has outlined a series of tasks that both parent and infant need to achieve in order to fulfil their developmental functions:

- *Attachment bonding*

  The baby has a desire to be near the carer in order to feel safe and secure while the parent feels closeness, love and affection for the baby which transcends place, time, demands and events.

- *Vigilance–protection*

  Babies are sensitive to changes in themselves and their environment. They will alert their carer when their comfort zones are exceeded, while parents feel a sense of responsibility to protect and maintain the safety and comfort of their baby.

- *Physiological regulation–providing structure*

  As babies grow, they become more able to regulate their own environment to make their needs known, but for this to happen the parent needs to be predictable and consistent in response to the baby's signals.

- *Affect regulation–empathic responsiveness*

  Babies feel strong emotions and the parent anticipates and monitors the baby's feelings so that they can be regulated. The parents must prioritise and respond to the needs of their baby rather than their own.

- *Learning–teaching*

  Babies are learning rapidly and exponentially, while the parent is the route for the baby to acquire knowledge and experience about the world, predictably and safely.

- *Play–play*

  Play is a mutual source of pleasure, learning and socialisation and deepens attachments.

- *Self control–discipline*

  As the baby starts to develop a sense of control over their own biological and emotional states, the parent gradually provides a structure that is consistent and familiar so that the baby can anticipate and conform to external expectations.

These stages demonstrate the depth of the interweaving and interdependency that is created in a loving and warm parent-infant relationship. However, when a parent has difficulty in feeling affection towards their baby, they also find difficulty in understanding the baby's needs. They are not alert to potential danger and threat, and are unable to help their baby manage their own feelings or the demands of the world. In extreme cases, this can result in physical and emotional neglect of the child, whereby the parent avoids the situation of caring for the child rather than confront their parenting difficulties. The stress and frustration of attempting to cope with the child in isolation can also result in physical assaults on the child, hence physical abuse and neglect are highly associated.

CHILD PROTECTION

Part of the role of every health professional providing services to families with young children is to be aware of and alert to possible child maltreatment. Even a decade ago, 1.5% of the 11 million children in England were subject to child protection inquiry for suspected child maltreatment. Approximately one-quarter of these children were then the subject of a child protection conference from which 15% were placed on the child protection register under the following definitions (Dept of Health, 1995). The definitions currently used in England and Wales for children placed on child protection registers (Dept of Health et al., 1999) include the following categories:

- Physical abuse may involve hitting, shaking, throwing, poisoning, burning or scalding, drowning, suffocating, or otherwise causing physical harm to a child. Physical harm may also be caused when a parent or carer feigns the symptoms of, or deliberately causes ill-health to a child whom they are looking after. This situation is commonly described using terms such as factitious illness by proxy or Munchausen syndrome by proxy.
- Emotional abuse is the persistent emotional ill-treatment of a child such as to cause severe and persistent adverse effects on the child's emotional development. It may involve conveying to children that they are worthless or unloved, inadequate, or valued only insofar as they meet the needs of another person. It may feature age or developmentally inappropriate expectations being imposed on children. It may involve causing children frequently to feel frightened or in danger, or the exploitation or corruption of children. Some level of emotional abuse is involved in all types of maltreatment of a child, though it may occur alone.
- Sexual abuse involves forcing or enticing a child or young person to take part in sexual activities whether or not the child is aware of what is

happening. The activities may involve physical contact including pene-trative (e.g., rape or buggery) or non-penetrative acts. They may include non-contact activities, such as involving children in looking at, or in the production of, pornographic material or watching sexual activities, or encouraging children to behave in sexually inappropriate ways.

- Neglect is the persistent failure to meet a child's basic physical and/or psychological needs, likely to result in the serious impairment of the child's health or development (including non-organic failure to thrive). It may involve a parent or carer failing to provide adequate food, shelter and clothing, failing to protect a child from physical harm or danger, or the failure to ensure access to appropriate medical care or treatment. It may also include neglect of, or unresponsiveness to, a child's basic emotional needs.

(From: *Working Together to Safeguard Children*,
Department of Health et al., 1999, pp. 5–6)

All the above definitions are used to consider child maltreatment perpe-trated by family members or by someone outside the child's home or extended family. During a child protection conference, mixed categories may be acknowledged where the child is suffering more than one type of abuse and/or neglect at the same time.

Although it is the statutory duty of police and social services to jointly investigate allegations of child maltreatment 'where there is reasonable cause to suspect that a child is suffering, or likely to suffer, significant harm', there is a clear expectation that doctors and nurses must refer their concerns to these statutory agencies (Dept of Health et al., 1999). It is generally con-sidered that withholding information about on-going child maltreatment, even on the basis of patient confidentiality, is professional malpractice: 'all health service staff have a duty to protect children' (Dept of Health, 1996). Therefore, an established multi-disciplinary network for consultation and referral is essential in any child protection system.

THE CHILD ASSESSMENT RATING AND EVALUATION PROGRAMME (CARE)

The CARE programme (Browne, Hamilton & Ware, 1995) was developed in response to a need for community health workers (including health visitors, midwives and community physicians) to be aware of and assess more accu-rately the emotional needs of all families with babies under the age of one year. The overall aim was the prevention of child abuse and neglect before it starts.

The Framework of the Assessment of Children in Need and their Families (Dept of Health et al., 2000) specifies that 'local authority and health authorities have a duty to safeguard and promote the welfare of children in their area who are in need' (p. viii). Safeguarding has two elements:

- a duty to protect children from maltreatment
- a duty to prevent impairment.

Promoting welfare creates opportunities for children to have optimum life chances in adulthood and ensure that they grow up in the context of safe and effective care. However, assessing children in need does create a necessity for clarity about the respective roles of each professional involved in the assessment and requires professionals to be clear about how information will be recorded and shared across professional boundaries and within agencies.

The CARE programme incorporates all of the principles underlying assessment of children in need (Dept of Health et al., 2000, p. 10), which requires that assessments:

- are child centred
- are rooted in child development
- are ecological in their approach
- ensure equality of opportunity
- involve working with children and families
- build on strengths as well as identify difficulties
- are inter-agency in their approach to assessment and the provision of services
- are a continuing process
- are not a single event
- are carried out in parallel with other action and providing services
- are grounded in evidence-based knowledge.

The competency framework (Dept of Health et al., 2004e) reaffirms the view that health visitors are expected to consider the parent(s) social and emotional wellbeing and take account of the quality and nature of social support networks and the impact of the transition to parenthood. The CARE programme provides an assessment package that enables community nurses to address these issues and the quality of the parent/child relationship with their baby, so that services reach the families most in need and, in doing so, even out inequalities of opportunity. The focus is on developing a partnership with parents and, where necessary, to empower them to identify solutions to their problems.

CARE is a home visiting programme for all families in the community during the infant's first year of life. It is a child centred assessment of need and development that is undertaken in partnership with parents, providing parents with a means of identifying their own situation and perceptions of parenthood in conjunction with a health professional. The CARE programme also provides health visitors and midwives with a tool that produces a more objective assessment procedure that can link effectively to 'need, risk or significant harm' assessments.

However, the CARE programme is not just an assessment procedure. As well as involving families in deciding their own needs for support, it provides an inclusive approach to record keeping and caseload management for professionals. It provides guidance on recording information so that it is accessible for professionals and safe for families. The structured caseload management system creates ease of communication, a uniform approach in collecting data across whole districts and identifies the agreed categories of work that health visitors can effectively engage with and have recognisable health gain outcome based upon evidence-based practice. The CARE programme incorporates two major facets of observation:

- The Index of Need – undertaken in partnership with parents.
- The assessment of indicators of infant attachment – utilising infant and parental observations.

PRACTICAL IMPLEMENTATION OF THE CARE PROGRAMME

The CARE programme approach can be incorporated into the normal health-visiting pattern used in the community during which public health considerations are discussed. It has been used and assessed in the context of health visiting programmes in the first year of life but part of it is equally applicable for use by midwives during contact with mothers during pregnancy. The key features include a planned visiting framework during which the community health worker can assess the infant's emotional development and help the parents express their own feelings, concerns and worries about parenting and their infant. For professionals, it offers reliable behavioural indicators to distinguish between priority cases and the remainder of the caseload.

Table 2.1 shows the outline of community nurse visits during the first year of a child's life. This is then outlined in more detail below, with the CARE components highlighted in italics. The 'Looking at your needs' booklet can be given to parents by midwives (see Appendix 1) or health visitors (see Appendix 2).

Table 2.1 Outline of the CARE programme in the first year of life

Newborn assessment (10–15 days)

1. Establishing initial contact
2. Baseline assessment of health needs of infant
3. Assessing family health needs
4. Observing social and home environment
5. Introducing parent held record
6. Promoting primary prevention
7. Introducing 'Looking at your Needs' Booklet
8. Forming aims for future visiting plan
9. Promoting attendance at Child Health Clinic

Home visit (4–6 weeks)

1. Reviewing 'Looking at your Needs' Booklet and Index of Need score
2. Identifying any implications of the Index of Need
3. Promoting health needs of child
4. Observing and discussing infant attachment behaviours and well being
5. Observing and discussing parental behaviour to infant
6. Edinburgh Postnatal Depression score (Cox et al., 1987)
7. Identifying additional services required

Home visit (3–5 months)

1. Discussing Index of Need results
2. Assessing infant's developmental progress
3. Promoting health needs of child, i.e., immunisations, diet, accident prevention, dental care
4. Assessing family health needs
5. Assessing mother's postnatal mental health
6. Observing and discussing infant attachment behaviours and well being
7. Observing and discussing parental behaviour to infant
8. Identifying additional services required
9. Reviewing additional services provided

Clinic assessment (7–9 months)

1. Developmental assessment and hearing test of infant
2. Observing and discussing infant attachment behaviours
3. Observing and discussing parental behaviour towards infant
4. Reviewing services needed and provided
5. Home visit for non-attenders

Home visit (12 months)

1. Final public health assessment
2. Final observation of infant attachment behaviours
3. Final observation of parent behaviour towards infant
4. Review of services provided and needed in the future
5. Overall rating of psychological care of the child
6. Child welfare factors at end of first year
7. Parent's sensitivity to child at end of first year
8. Assessment of priority and future caseload category

Newborn Assessment (10–15 Days After Birth)

(i)   Establish initial contact. This first home visit after birth should be a relaxed introductory session that usually takes about one hour. The parent is assessing her feelings about the health visitor as well as the health visitor gaining first impressions about the parents. This visit commences the start of the parent partnership approach where both parent and professional work together to develop their aims and discuss their observations. It is also a time for parents to discuss their concerns.

(ii)   A baseline assessment of the health status and health needs of the infant should be conducted and there may be a basic examination of the baby (e.g., weighing and measuring).

(iii)   An assessment of family health needs should also be conducted and basic socio-demographic information recorded. There can be:
   • discussion of the mother's recovery from the birth
   • discussion of the general welfare of the parents
   • information about the parent(s) health.

(iv)   Observation of the social and home environment of the baby and the parents. This includes:
   • the other demands on the parents
   • the level of deprivation in the area
   • signs of stress due to external environment, i.e., housing conditions
   • financial problems
   • home management
   • accessibility of home with a baby
   • neighbours
   • social isolation
   • pets
   • demands of other children.

(v)   The parent-held record should be given to the parent(s) and discussed, drawing particular attention to the colour coded section on Emotional Development, which is used as the basis for discussion about the baby's emotional development throughout the first year.

(vi)   Primary prevention should be promoted through:
   • information about clinics and community groups
   • advice about baby care if required
   • discussion about immunisations.

(vii)   The concept of the CARE programme should be discussed and the 'Looking at your Needs' booklet about the CARE programme given to the parents (see Appendices 1 and 2). This includes showing the Index of Need to parents (see Chapter 3 & Appendix 3, page 169) and inviting them to think about it before the next visit.

(viii) The aims for a future visiting plan should be established. If the health visitor detects problems then early or more regular visiting may be agreed with the parents.

(ix) Promotion of attendance at Child Health Clinic. The health visitor will provide her address and telephone number at the local clinic and details on how to reach the clinic. The parents should be invited to attend the clinic regularly to weigh the baby or discuss any concerns that they have and given information about support and advice they can receive.

The aim of this primary home visit is to answer the following questions:

1. How can I help these parents? What do they need?
2. Can they manage on their own?
3. Are they being honest with me? Can I believe what they say?
4. Is this baby safe? Will this baby stay safe?
5. Can these parents cope with providing the essentials to ensure the baby thrives, i.e., food, warmth, stimulation and protection?

Planned Home Visit (4–6 Weeks of Life)

Mothers have usually recovered from the birth both emotionally and physically by this stage and if this is not the case then the effect will be noticeable. Postnatal depression, in particular, can be evident while it may not have been so apparent at the primary visit. The parents also now understand through experience what the impact of the new baby really means in terms of life changes. They can at times feel resentful and depressed.

(i) The 'Looking at your Needs' booklet should be discussed and parents asked whether they have had time to look at it. The Index of Need score should also be discussed. The parents can often reflect on their own perceived needs at this stage. The psychosocial impact of the new baby on the parents can be explored with them.

(ii) Any implications from the Index of Need should be identified together with the parents and additional services or need for resources can be planned. Some parents may wish to take time to discuss issues in their history that this has raised. Also, parents may raise fears and worries about their own ability to parent effectively or discuss concerns about existing emotional difficulties in the parental or family relationships (Appendix 3, page 171).

(iii) The health needs of the infant should be discussed with the parents. The baby will be changing and signs of physical development can be talked about. The weight of the baby, the baby's appetite and changes in the pattern of breast or bottle-feeding are all important issues. The infant will be having a developmental assessment and a cardio-vascular assessment by the GP at this time along with the mother's six-week postnatal examination.

(iv) Specific public health topics are addressed with the parents, e.g.:
- accident prevention
- immunisation
- emotional health
- environmental factors such as infant nutrition
- the baby's changing developmental requirements
- the parents are encouraged to continue to attend the child health clinic.

(v) Sections of Form A related to the 4–6 week visit (see Appendix 3, pages 170–170) should be completed. This includes:
- Observing and discussing indicators of the infant's attachment-forming behaviour towards the primary care-giver. Aspects of the baby's attachment-formation behaviour can be pointed out to the parents so that they understand their baby's behaviour and start to recognise the positive side of the attachment process. This opportunity can be taken to discuss age appropriate stimu-lation and play with the baby (see Appendix 3, page 172).
- Observing the parents' behaviour and attributions about their infant: parents will be able to discuss what their baby is like, as well as the effect of having a child on them and their lifestyle. The quality of their parenting style can start to be observed (see Appen-dix 3, page 172).

(vi) An Edinburgh Postnatal Depression Score (Cox et al., 1987) should be obtained in order to assess the impact of the birth on the mother's mental health. A score of 12 or more indicates the likelihood of post-natal depression, although this should not overrule clinical judgement. Issues about support required by the mother can then be identified early on before a crisis occurs.

(vii) Appropriate resources can be mobilised to address the identified areas of need within the CARE programme.

The aim of this visit is to answer the following questions:

1. Is this a baby who requires priority of resources?
2. Is this a child at risk of significant harm?
3. What type of support does this family require in order to achieve 'good enough parenting' so that the infant can have his/her rights met to grow and reach his/her full potential?
4. Are public health needs being addressed?

5. Is the infant making normal developmental progress?
6. Is this mother showing any signs of postnatal depression?

Planned Home Visit (3–5 Months of Life)

This visit enables parents to think about their role as parents and they often raise issues that they may not have been able to discuss earlier or that they find will not go away. This planned visit is one that seems to prevent crisis interventions later.

(i)   The issues raised by the Index of Need may still require discussion or may even be raised for the first time (if it has not been possible before) now that the parents have become familiar with their health visitor (see Appendix 3, page 173).

(ii)   A developmental assessment of the infant should be undertaken and opportunities provided to the parents to discuss how to promote the baby's developmental progress. The parents should also learn about the capabilities of their infant and what to look out for.

(iii)   Areas of public health promotion that should be discussed include:
   • first and second immunisations
   • the infant's weaning and dietary requirements
   • dentition and dental health
   • accident prevention
   • evaluation of the family health needs.

(iv)   Assessment of family health needs should be continued and a discussion to stimulate awareness of community activities (including those of child minding and issues related to parents' return to work) can be important at this time.

(v)   An assessment of the mother's postnatal emotional and mental health is important at this stage after birth.

(vi)   The remainder of Form A (see Appendix 3, page 173) related to the 3–4 month visit should be completed. This will include:
   • Observation of indicators of attachment-forming behaviour which the infant displays towards the primary care-giver and is indicative of the infant's emotional development (see Appendix 3, page 173).
   • Observation of the parents' attributions about their infant, their perceptions of their infant and the quality of parenting (see Appendix 3, page 173).

(vii)   Appropriate resources should be mobilised to address the identified areas of need within the CARE programme.

(viii) There should also be a review of any additional resources that the family have used and whether they have been effective and should continue.

The aim of this visit is to answer the following questions:

1. Is this parent adapting to and understanding the needs of the infant?
2. Is this baby safe?
3. Are appropriate care arrangements in place if mother wants to return to work?
4. Is this baby showing signs of appropriate attachment-formation behaviour to the primary carer?
5. Is this mother receiving support within the community? Is she socially isolated?
6. Is this mother showing signs of postnatal depression?
7. Are the parents making positive comments about their infant?
8. Does this family require any additional services?

Planned Clinic Visit (7–9 Months of Life)

This assessment is incorporated into the health promotion programme and is undertaken at the clinic, with a home visit for non-attenders.

(i)   The public health tasks at this visit include a developmental assessment and a Distraction Hearing Test.
(ii) Form B of the CARE programme that relates to the 7–9 month visit (see Appendix 4, pages 176–177) should be completed. This includes:
   • Observation of indicators of attachment behaviour which the infant displays towards the primary care-giver and is indicative of the infant's emotional development.
   • Observation of the parents' attributions about their infant, their perceptions of their infant and the quality of parenting using the Observation of Parenting Style. Observation is possible during the administering of the developmental tests where the baby is exposed to a stranger and can be comforted by the mother.
(iii) This session also provides an opportunity for a preliminary evaluation of initial intervention and any remedial action taken with the family. Consideration can be given to whether the infant or family will require further intervention beyond the age of one year. Changes in family circumstances should be recorded.

The aim of this visit is to answer the following questions:

1. If the family have been attending any additional services how effective has this been? Do they require further or different help and support?
2. Is the baby making appropriate emotional and developmental progress?

3. Are alternative care arrangements safe for the child and meeting the child's emotional and developmental needs?
4. Are the parents showing any emotional or mental health problems?
5. Is the baby safe? Is a home visit required?
6. Have all of the public health issues been addressed?

Planned Home Visit (12 Months of Life)

This visit is designed to complete the assessment of 'priority' for this infant that has been developing during the course of the year. A judgement will be made about the infant's needs and the level of subsequent service to the family beyond the age of one year.

(i) The public health final assessment includes:
- discussions around accident prevention
- child protection
- family health education
- continued community support system
- the services available in the area
- informing parents about how to contact their health visitor if they require services over the next 18 months
- informing parents of the further developmental assessment due at age 2–2.5 years.

(ii) The final assessment of the CARE programme through completion of Form B relating to the 12 month visit (see Appendix 4, pages 178–179). This includes:
  a. A further discussion of the Index of Need with the parents to determine if they want to amend any details or report changes that have occurred over the course of the year (see Appendix 4, page 178).
  b. Observing the parenting style to note the parents' attributions, perceptions of the infant and the quality of parenting (see Appendix 4, page 179).
  c. A final assessment of the indicators of the quality of attachment of the infant to the primary care-giver. This should include a clear understanding of whether the infant is being observed in its familiar surroundings, whether the care-giver is relaxed or whether there are apparent stress factors overriding the situation. The observation should be made in the context of the previous observations throughout the year (see Appendix 4, pages 177 and 179).
  d. A report should also be made on the family in relation to welfare factors such as safety, feeding, accommodation, cleanliness, appearance and clothing of the child (see Appendix 4, page 180).

e. The parent's sensitivity to the child should be observed and recorded, i.e., prompt responsiveness, appropriate responses, consistent responses and smooth, sensitive interaction with the infant (see Appendix 4, page 181).

f. An overall rating of psychological care of the child is provided including affection, security, guidance and control, independence and stimulation of the infant (see Appendix 4, page 182). These parameters of observation can easily be incorporated into the professional record, thus reducing additional paperwork.

g. In consultation with the family, the health visitor should record all of the referrals made for the family over the past 12 months and the total number of visits made to them (see Appendix 4, page 183). There are a number of potential referrals to other agencies (see Table 2.2)

h. On the basis of observations and Index of Need a decision should be made about the level of need for the family (see Appendix 4, page 183). This should be a culmination of the observation over the first year and will lead the health visitor to judge whether the case can be classified as:

   (i) Inactive routine caseload where the assessment has not identified any concerns and the infant has attained normal physical and emotional development.

   (ii) Selective caseload where a prolonged intervention programme will be required after the first year of life. The Selective caseload has the following categories:

   • Children on the Child Protection Register
   • Children classified as 'In Need' referred to Social services
   • Children with a significant Index of Need (five or over)
   • Children with a diagnosed disability or health need
   • Children with a developmental delay
   • Looked after children.

The aim of this visit is to answer the following questions:

1. Is this final observation a 'one off' situation or typical of what has been observed over the previous year?

2. If the family have been attending any additional services how effective has this been? What do they require in terms of further or different help and support?

3. What level of need does this family have? Can the case be safely designated to routine non-active caseload?

4. If the case is designated into the 'selective' caseload, in which category should they be placed?

5. What type of care plan is required if this case is kept 'active'?

6. What are the supervision areas the practitioner needs to discuss with their supervisor?

Table 2.2 Potential referrals by the community nurse for the child and the family during the first year after birth*

Referral agency	Type of support offered
Health Visiting Service	Groups for: postnatal depression, parental coping, infant sleep difficulties, infant feeding difficulties, individual counselling
Voluntary Groups	Home Start lay visitor scheme, mother and toddler community groups, family network groups, voluntary counselling service, Relate
Health Services	General Practitioner, paediatrician, child and family psychiatric service, adult mental health service, community psychiatric nurse service, psychology service
Social Care and Health Services (indirect referral to police services via social worker if necessary for child protection concerns)	Nursery placements, housing department, social care support for children in need, disability services (e.g., for respite care, support for parents), child protection social work, child protection conferences

* for any local area, this multi-sector referral network should be in place prior to any assessment of children and their families.

CHILDREN WHO TRANSFER INTO THE CARE PROGRAMME

Whilst ideally, all children in an area using the CARE programme would be included from birth, it is necessary to take account of those children who move into the area at some time during their first year. Such children can be easily transferred into the ongoing system. This occurs through the health visitor evaluating the 'hand over' from the transferring health visitor and establishing any identified needs. A home visit should then be made within **one week** of the transfer so that the health visitor can introduce herself to the family and introduce the Health Visiting Service. The Index of Need should be given to the parents at this visit and baseline assessment undertaken of the family health needs.

If the infant is under one year of age an agreement should be reached about:

- entering into the CARE programme assessment and home visiting structure
- undertaking the infant's developmental assessment in accordance with the programme
- following up the Index of Need with the family within **two weeks** of introducing it to the family
- opening the case within the Active caseload

If the child is over one year of age then an agreement should be reached about:

- arranging further contact in accordance with the quality standard time frames
- following up the Index of Need with the family within **two weeks** of introducing it
- informing the family about registering with a GP if they have not already done so
- informing the parents about local community services
- providing information about health clinics and 'drop in' services
- providing a seamless service with the assessment of the child that follows on from previous work in the transferring authority
- deciding whether the case should be allocated to the Selective, Inactive or Routine Caseload.

TRANSFER OF CHILDREN OUT OF THE CARE PROGRAMME

When a family moves within or out of the district or transfers to a new GP, the health visitor should follow their professional quality standards for the transfer of records and information to the new health authority and health visitor. Children and families who are on the CARE Programme will have a transfer of care that contains the following information in order to ensure continuity of service for the child and family:

- a synopsis of the assessment of need which has taken place to date
- the Index of Need characteristics if the score is 5 or above
- an evaluation of progress made whilst receiving the CARE programme
- an assessment of the behaviour observations
- an opinion of what follow-on services may be required
- information to other professional colleagues about the transfer so that they can liaise with their counterpart in the new authority
- a contact name, address and telephone number in case the receiving health visitor needs to clarify any information.

CONCLUSION

In order to fully understand the CARE programme, the main tenets of the child assessment rating and evaluation procedures need to be given in more detail in the following chapters with a description of the research evidence on which it was based.

3

THE INDEX OF NEED

Trying to identify and predict which families with babies and young children will need additional support and help during the early years is difficult. However, resources are often scarce and it is also important to target the resources that are available to the families that are most 'in need'. Prioritising services creates a situation where decisions need to be made by primary health care workers based on their knowledge and observations of the parents and infant.

SCREENING POPULATIONS USING A CHECKLIST APPROACH

One way of trying to decide which families need help is to look at the constellation of factors that exist in other families that are in distress or where children have been assessed as suffering significant harm. This provides a checklist of factors that have been found to be common in these families. These factors are only guidelines and do not provide an absolute watertight prediction. Risk factors can never be considered as sufficient causal explanations. There is a relatively low proportion of child abuse and neglect in the general population so a very large number of families need to be screened in order to find the few that are at risk. Failing to identify a child who is at risk of suffering significant harm may result in no intervention being provided and the child remaining unprotected from harm. But the opposite can also occur. Some children may be identified as being at risk of significant harm and services provided when in fact the family has been inappropriately labelled. Any screening or checklist approach has the risk of identifying false positives or false negatives (see Table 3.1).

The task of any predictive screening checklist is to try to achieve 100% true positives (sensitivity) and true negatives (specificity) and 0% false positives (false alarms) and false negatives (missed cases). However, this is generally not achievable. If the checklist's sensitivity is set too high then too

Table 3.1 Classification of children, parents or families following a screening procedure

True Positive	False Positive
accurate identification of risk of significant harm	inaccurately identified as a case at risk of significant harm
False Negative	**True Negative**
missed a case at risk of significant harm	accurate identification of no risk of significant harm

many cases will be missed, but if it is set too low then too many false positives will be identified. The sensitivity (i.e., the accurate prediction of cases at risk of significant harm) and the specificity (i.e., the accurate prediction of cases with no risk of significant harm) of the checklist need to be balanced in order to gain the best possible prediction. With child maltreatment being relatively rare in families, the positive predictive accuracy will rarely exceed 80% of cases (Agathonos & Browne, 1997).

When designing a checklist it is necessary to consider whether the number of items should just be added together as a total or whether certain items may be more predictive than others, therefore requiring a weighting to make them more important in the sum total. Weighting can help improve the sensitivity and specificity.

Browne & Saqi (1988a) evaluated a health visitor checklist of 12 risk factors that could be completed on one occasion (see Table 3.2). In Surrey, 14,238 births were screened: 949 (6.7%) of families were considered to be 'high risk' on the basis of the checklist. Within two years of birth, 6% of the high risk group had been referred for abuse or neglect of their child. Five years after birth, only 7.5% of the high risk group had been referred (Browne & Herbert, 1997). Therefore, the level of false positives was high. In addition, 0.2% of the 'low risk' families abused their child within the first two years after birth, marginally rising to 0.26% five years after birth (see Figure 3.1).

Follow-up at five years, found that 106 (11%) of the families had attended a case conference for suspected or actual maltreatment of their newborn infant (Browne & Herbert, 1997). The 12-item checklist was 'sensitive' to 72 (68%) of the cases (hits), but 34 (32%) had been missed (i.e., false negatives). The checklist also correctly 'specified' 13,254 (94%) low-risk families who did not go on to abuse their children, but raised a false alarm with 892 (6.3%) families who were incorrectly classified as high risk (false positives). Nearly one-third (32%) of the abusing families were missed and identified as 'low risk' around the time of birth (false negatives) but went on to be referred for child maltreatment within five years of birth.

Table 3.2 Relative predictive values of screening characteristics for child abuse
(from Browne & Herbert, 1997, p. 121)

Checklist characteristics	Abusing families (%) (n = 106)	Non-abusing families (%) (n = 14,146)	Conditional probability* (%) 0.7
History of family violence	30.2	1.6	12.4
Parent indifferent, intolerant or over-anxious towards child	31.1	3.1	7.0
Single or separated parent	48.1	6.9	5.0
Socio-economic problems, e.g., unemployment	70.8	12.9	3.9
History of mental illness, drug or alcohol addiction	34.9	4.8	5.2
Parent abused or neglected as a child	19.8	1.8	7.6
Infant premature, low birth weight	21.7	6.9	2.3
Infant separated from mother for more than 24 hours post delivery	12.3	3.2	2.8
Mother less than 21 years old at time of birth	29.2	7.7	2.8
Step parent or cohabitee present	27.4	6.2	3.2
Less than 18 months between birth of children	16.0	7.5	1.6
Infant mentally or physically handicapped	2.8	1.1	1.9

* (Conditional probability refers to the percentage of families with a particular characteristic that will later abuse and/or neglect their newborn in the first five years of life.)

Pragmatically, the use of this checklist alone, would result in the health visitor trying to identify the one potential maltreating family within every 13 cases classified as high risk. Even more problematic is the identification of the 'missed' cases amongst the low risk population (one in every 391 families). Without the use of the checklist, the health visitor needs to consider the possibility of one maltreating family in every 134 families with a newborn baby. Hence, the checklist is of some use but needs further sophistication to distinguish the true cases from the false cases. It was therefore recognised that additional screening approaches would be required in addition to the checklist.

Table 3.2 (above) identifies the importance of the different risk factors in predicting child abuse and, as can be seen, no single factor is sufficiently predictive in isolation to identify abusive situations in a family. In fact, the

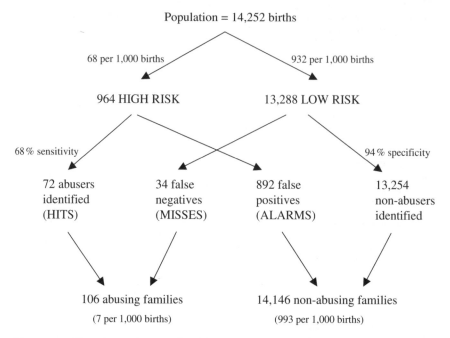

Figure 3.1 Use of a twelve-item health visitor checklist in Surrey to screen for potential of significant harm in families with newborns who were then followed up for five years to determine outcome (adapted from Browne & Herbert, 1997)

conditional probability of any single factor being predictive is very low. We can try to increase the rate of predictability by:

• rating a group of factors that occur together
• carrying out on-going assessment during the first year of life as family circumstances change rather than having a one point assessment
• carrying out additional observations of parent-child interaction to assess the level of parenting skills and attachment/attitude to the infant.

RISK FACTORS ASSOCIATED WITH SIGNIFICANT HARM FOR CHILDREN

Research indicates that a number of characteristics associated with the child, the parent, the family and the community are associated with child abuse and neglect (Ammerman & Hersen, 1990, 1992). The prevalence of these so-called 'risk' factors is above that considered to be average for the population as a whole (Newcomb & Locke, 2001; Pears & Capaldi, 2001).

These situational risk factors can either remain static or change in a family over time. Static risk factors are those past experiences that cannot be changed, yet may affect the current way a parent cares for his/her child (e.g., mother less than 21 years at time of birth). In contrast, dynamic risk factors are those that are able to change with intervention and/or support (e.g., parent indifferent, intolerant or over-anxious towards child). In addition, changing relationships between parents, marital breakdown and new cohabitees are all significant events that can affect the parents emotional state and the infant. Thus, the causes of significant harm that children may experience are multi-factorial and complex. This is because the factors at each level interact to increase or decrease the chances of maltreatment occurring in the family. These levels are typically categorised as those relating to the child, the parent, the family and the community (Bronfenbrenner, 1979; Hamilton & Browne, 2002). Societal values may also influence the prevalence of these factors. Risk factors for the potential for child maltreatment are as follows:

- Child characteristics include temperamental characteristics, physical health and disability, prematurity, unwanted child, low birth-weight and complications at birth.
- Parent characteristics include parenting skills, mental and physical health/disability, substance misuse, immature age, physically or sexually abused as a child, and biologically unrelated to child.
- Family characteristics include marital discord, single parenting, uncommitted cohabitees, social isolation, serious financial difficulties and birth spacings (e.g., twins).
- Community characteristics include the demographic and cultural situation of the community (e.g., high crime area), level of poverty and unemployment.

Parents or carers may have clearly defined harmful attributes and these should be viewed seriously in the context of child care. However, even though one parent may suffer considerable difficulties there may be another parent who is able to provide protection and nurturing to the infant. One of the highest risks is when there is a single parent with these serious difficulties coping alone with their infant.

STATIC RISK FACTORS

Complications during Birth

Abnormal pregnancy, labour and delivery, and separation of the baby from the mother at birth have been observed to have a higher prevalence amongst parents who abuse their children (Brown et al., 1998; Lynch, 1975). The extra stress associated with caring for a sick child or a child with growth difficulties has also been associated with maltreatment (Iwaniec, 2004).

Premature, Low-birth-weight Child

A number of researchers report a higher prematurity rate and low birth weights amongst abused or neglected children ranging from 13–30% (see Browne & Saqi, 1988a). This may partly be because of their less attractive appearance and the fact that their cries are perceived to be more piercing and aversive compared to full-term births (Frodi & Lamb, 1980).

Child with Physical or Intellectual Disability

The number of children with disabilities among maltreating families is twice that observed in the general population. It is difficult to ascertain in these samples whether the abuse and/or neglect have occurred as a result of the disability or whether the disability was caused by the maltreatment (Browne & Saqi, 1988a; Goldson, 1998; Morgan, 1987).

Birth Spacing (Less than 18 Months between Births or Twins)

Larger family size has been found to be associated with maltreating families (Belsky, 1993), but so too have families with twins (Nelson & Martin, 1985). Therefore, spacing between births may be more important than the number of children in the family due to the increased stress of having more than one completely dependent and demanding child. Of course, families can only achieve large numbers of children with relatively small spacing between births.

Parent not Biologically Related to Child

The relationship between step-parenting and child maltreatment is well-established (Finkelhor et al., 1990; Giles-Sims & Finkelhor, 1984). Studies demonstrate that a step-parent was living in the family home in 15% of all maltreatment cases, 25% of non-accidental injury cases and 43% of fatalities (Wilson & Daly, 1987). In a sample of English police child protection units, it was shown that although the step-father was the perpetrator in 11% of all maltreatment cases referred, when only those children living with a step-father were considered, it rose to 53% (Hamilton & Browne, 1999).

Parent Has a History of Mental Health Difficulties

Glaser & Prior (1997) reviewed the cases of all children whose names were on the Child Protection Registers of four English local authorities. Parental mental illness, including suicide attempts, anorexia nervosa, depressive psychosis and schizophrenia was present in 31% of cases. The prevalence of these disorders in parents of children on the register was considerably higher than in the general population where rates for mental illness have been estimated at 15% for depression (Kandal et al., 1991) and just under 1% for schizophrenia (Bamrah et al., 1991). Thus, Briere (1992) concludes that parental mental health difficulties are highly associated with child trauma.

The effect of parental psychiatric disorder on children's psychological welfare and development was determined by the social and relational consequences of the parent's disorders (Quinton & Rutter, 1984). It is the manifestation of the parent's problems through their behaviour that creates the risk to their children. A parent who is self-preoccupied or emotionally and practically unavailable as the result of a mental health problem is more likely to neglect their children than those who show unpredictable or chaotic forward planning due to psychosis or depression. Physical abuse is more likely to result from parental irritability or over-reaction to stresses that often accompany anxiety, depression or psychosis than the parent's distorted beliefs or aggressive behaviour during psychotic episodes (Reder & Duncan, 2000).

The death of a child through abuse also shows an association with parental mental health problems. A review of 48 children's deaths in England indicated that 50% of parents suffered from a current psychiatric disorder, 48% had previously received psychiatric treatment, 31% had made a prior suicide attempt, 24% were diagnosed as depressed and 24% diagnosed as psychotic at the time of the killing (Wilczynski, 1997). Reder and Duncan (1999b) also reviewed 35 cases of child death and found that 43% of the care-givers had been suffering from an active mental health problem at the time they killed the child.

Parent under 21 Years at Birth of Child

Parents who are very young or who have learning difficulties may experience significant problems in the complex decision making that occurs in caring for a baby and they may have limited awareness of their baby's needs or a limited ability to solve problems. Thus, younger parents have also been associated with higher risk of child maltreatment (Egeland et al., 2002; Straus, 1994).

Parent Has a History of Physical or Sexual Abuse as a Child

The consensus from research is that individuals with a history of abuse in childhood are at increased risk of maltreating their own children (Buchanan, 1996; Egeland, Bosquet & Chung, 2002). However, this intergenerational pathway of maltreatment is not inevitable and is the result of a complex interaction between risk, protective and mediating factors (Dixon, Browne & Hamilton-Giachritsis, 2005; Dixon, Hamilton-Giachritsis & Browne, 2005). For example, the static risk factor of young parental age in parents abused as a child interacts with dynamic risk factors such as a higher probability of living with a violent adult, which facilitates the intergenerational cycle (Fantuzzo et al., 1997; Tajima, 2000) or increased social support (i.e., a lack of social isolation) which may break the cycle. These various pathways have a strong influence on the attributions and behaviours of parents towards their child and the parenting style adopted (Dixon, Hamilton-Giachritsis & Browne, 2005).

Parents may have unresolved feelings and problems related to their own past experiences or childhood when they may have experienced abuse or neglect. These feelings are resurrected when they become parents them-selves and painful memories can interfere with their ability to parent effec-tively or safely. They may have difficulty in recognising positive behaviours in their infant and have problems delivering consistent positive parenting. They may not model positive or appropriate social behaviours themselves and fail to notice or affirm it in their infant. They may find it difficult to recognise their infant as an individual with a separate identity and differing needs. The process of teaching their child to anticipate consequences or problem solve may be very difficult for parents who struggle to reflect on their own impulsive responses. An absence of early models of good parent-ing experiences for themselves may compromise their understanding of the child's age appropriate emotional needs and the level of protection required. To be able to understand the tasks of parenting, adults need to be able to make links with their own childhood experiences and reflect on the parent-ing they received, but this is extremely difficult if those experiences were rejecting or abusive (Westman, 2000).

Often adverse experiences in childhood are associated with adult psycho-pathology or personality disorders, which can create poor parenting experi-ences for infants (Reder & Duncan, 1999a). Personality disorders can result in deliberate self-harm, interpersonal conflict and domestic violence; all of which have serious consequences for the child, either as an extension of this personal violence or as a witness to it.

DYNAMIC RISK FACTORS

Current Mental Health Difficulties

Depression has been highlighted as one of the most prevalent mental health problems in parents with young children. It is highly prevalent in child-bearing women with approximately 8 % of mothers being clinically depressed at any one time (Downey & Coyne, 1990).

The incidence of postnatal depression is approximately 10–15 % of mothers during the first year following birth and its onset is typically in the first three months after delivery, sometimes lasting for six months or up to a year if left untreated (Cooper et al., 1988; Oates, 1994). Maternal postnatal depression can be significantly harmful to young infants particularly between the ages of 6 and 18 months of age, with an increased incidence of insecure attachment in 18-month-old infants (Murray, 1992; Murray & Cooper, 1996). The depression itself does not cause the difficulties in the infant; it is the effect on the mother-child interaction that does the damage. This may lead to longer term changes in children's behaviour and emotional state, including social withdrawal, negativity and distress (Dawson et al., 1994) and also effects on emotional and cognitive development (Hay et al., 2001).

Pregnancy and the post partum period are risk periods for the development and exacerbation of anxiety disorders. Therefore, new mothers may be faced with the distress and impact of an anxiety disorder at the time when their preoccupation and energy need to be directed towards the baby in order to facilitate the development of a warm, secure and responsive relationship (Fellow-Smith, 2000). Panic attacks, obsessive-compulsive disorder and agoraphobia can all disrupt the parenting style of the mother and the consequent attachment of the infant. One study has shown the rate of insecure attachment in the children of parents with anxiety disorders to be as high as 80 % (Manassis et al., 1995).

Women in the post partum period also have a greater risk of becoming psychotic, admission to psychiatric hospital, and/or psychiatric referral in general, than at any other time in their lives (Etchegoyen, 2000). The problems faced by women and their babies during the perinatal period present the health services with a demand for an effective and cooperative interface between adult and child mental health services, primary health care services and social services.

Nevertheless, it is important to remember that many parents with mental health problems can parent very effectively and make great efforts to ensure their child is not affected. Any assessment of the parental mental health status should include a diagnosis of the condition but also provide a detailed appraisal of the child's experiences of the parent's behaviour. Sometimes, though, there is failure to differentiate between the mother's needs as a patient, her needs as a parent and the child's needs. There may be some difficulties where the adult mental health professionals consider it is their responsibility to guard their patient's confidentiality even if this compromises the child's safety, but it is a principle of good practice to prioritise the child's welfare even if this means breaking confidentiality (Reder & Duncan, 2000). In general, if the child's needs are being met appropriately by the parents and their care arrangements, then there would not be cause for concern. Parents need to feel that the health care professionals are there to support them in their role and help them cope with difficulties that they might be having.

Parent Has a Dependency on Drugs or Alcohol

Glaser & Prior (1997) found that substance misuse was present in 26% of the child protection cases in four English health authorities, while the prevalence of parents in the general population who drink harmful levels of alcohol is 7% (Brisby et al., 1997). Studies of serious child abuse and/or neglect brought before the courts have found that a documented history of problems with alcohol or drugs was present in at least one parent in 43% of cases and this rose to 50% if suspicions of substance abuse were included (Murphy et al., 1991). Reder & Duncan's (1999b) study of fatal child abuse also found that 60% of the perpetrators had previously used substances immediately before the crime. Typically, substance-misusing parents' lifestyles were very self-centred and associated with a lack of supervision and neglect of the child. Some young children died after accidentally ingesting their parent's drugs found in the home. Furthermore, some parents may use their own substances to quieten a crying infant or toddler with normal challenging behaviour (Drummond & Fitzpatrick, 2000).

The risk factor of alcohol and drug dependency is often associated with other risk factors. There are increased rates of domestic violence, poverty and unemployment in families where the parents misuse alcohol or substances (Gullotta, Hampton & Jenkins, 1996; Hampton, Senatore & Gullotta, 1998; Hampton, 1999). *Alcohol* abuse may be more episodic and binge drinking may alternate with times when the parent is stable and loving. It also tends to be confined to one parent (Roberts, 1987). In contrast, parents who use *drugs* tend to show a more chaotic lifestyle and their misuse is more likely to be associated with criminal activity, with a tendency for both parents to be users. It appears to be the lifestyle associated with the substance abuse that impacts so severely on child care, rather than the drug use per se.

Parents who comply with drug treatment programmes appear to demonstrate better child caring capabilities than those who default (Reder & Duncan, 1999a). Swadi (1994) has outlined an assessment scheme for assessing the parenting skills of substance abusing parents. Apart from observing the accommodation, home environment and the provision of basic necessities, there are differing elements to assess which include the pattern of parental substance misuse, e.g.:

- Type, frequency, quantity and method of administration of the substances.
- Whether the misuse is stable or chaotic or involves swings between severe intoxication and withdrawal.
- Whether the parent is injecting and how this is managed in the home (is the child exposed to risk?).
- Child care arrangements while the parent is under the influence of the drugs?
- Is it in front of the child?
- Understanding of the effects of the substance misuse on the parental mental state and impact on their ability to care for the child.
- How the substances are procured (are the children left unattended, does the procurement take priority over spending time with the child?).
- The parent's perception of the situation, insight into what is happening and how realistic they are in their assessment of the effects on their child.
- The parent's motivation for change, which is a key element for treatment compliance (Prochaska & DiClemente, 1984).

One of the main problems of substance misuse is the association with all forms of family violence (Browne & Herbert, 1997): 60% of the partners of battered women have been shown to have an alcohol problem, while 21% have a drug problem (Roberts, 1987). Alcohol also significantly depresses adults' internal inhibitors and therefore may place children at greater risk of sexual abuse (Drummond & Fitzpatrick, 2000).

Violent Adult in the Family

Domestic violence (spouse abuse) has two main adverse effects on children. Firstly, it is an important predictor of child abuse and, secondly, it is related to adverse behavioural and emotional outcomes in the child (Browne & Herbert, 1997). Family violence is often associated with stress in the family and in the presence of poor and/or insecure relationships, this stress in family functioning can increase the likelihood of aggression in the family (Abidin, 1990; Browne & Herbert, 1997). There is a link between wife abuse and child abuse (Browne & Hamilton, 1999; Browne, Falshaw & Dixon, 2002) and the knowledge about violence in the family should alert health professionals to the increased possibility of the child being at risk. The risk of abuse to the child associated with living with violent parents is between three and nine times higher than in families where there is no violence (Moffit & Caspi, 1998). In addition, it has been shown that the severity of injury to both the mother and the child is greater where both spouse abuse and child abuse co-exist in the family (Browne & Hamilton, 1999).

If the parents have a violent relationship then it is likely that the child will witness violence between them at some time and find the experience traumatic (Jaffe, Wolfe & Wilson, 1990). It is therefore highly likely that the existence of a physically violent relationship between parents is associated with emotional abuse in the infant. Sometimes this emotional disturbance is characterised by hyperactivity in the child, which is then often identified by the parent as a conduct disorder or attention hyperactivity deficit disorder, which may be followed by inappropriate medication.

The peak rates for victimisation from spouse abuse coincide with the peak age for childbearing (i.e., 17–30 for women) so that high rates of spouse abuse are often observed in pregnant women. In a study of 290 pregnant women, Helton (1986) found that 15.2% reported battering before their current pregnancies and 8.3% during their current pregnancy. Therefore, for health professionals supporting pregnant women it is very important for them to consider the possibility of spouse abuse, especially as it has potentially dangerous consequences for the unborn child (McFarlane, 1991; Newberger et al., 1992). Pregnant women who receive an injury to their abdomen can experience miscarriage through the death of the foetus or detachment of the placenta. Furthermore, there is an increased risk of disability to the unborn child.

Non-marital cohabitation has higher rates of partner violence compared to married couples, being most common among partners with young children (Moffit & Caspi, 1998). Greater frequency and intensity of parental conflict is consistently associated with worse behaviour outcomes for the children, with physical violence being worse than mental and verbal conflict (Grynch & Fincham, 1990). Exposure to domestic violence is a risk factor in children for later development of anxiety, conduct disorders, criminal behaviour and problems with alcohol (Fergusson & Harwood, 1998).

Parent Feels Socially Isolated

Having a new baby may have a deleterious effect on the parent's emotional wellbeing and their relationship as a couple may be challenged. Those couples with already impoverished relationships may begin to feel emotion-ally isolated and neglected by their partner and this may be a trigger for relationship problems (Johnston & Campbell, 1988; McAllister, 1995).

Both parents may feel socially isolated or perceive a lack of social support from their family and friends. This social isolation has been associated with a greater probability of child abuse and/or neglect (Crouch, Milner & Thomsen, 2001; Egeland et al., 2002; Runtz & Shallow, 1997). Indeed, social support can act as a protective factor for parents abused and/or neglected as children and may help break the cycle of violence (Dixon, Browne & Hamilton-Giachritsis, in submission). However, the relationship between child abuse and social isolation is complex. The *quality* of social supports is considered to be more important to parents than the actual *quantity* (Seagull, 1987). Nevertheless, befriending and lay visitor schemes for parents at risk have had some success in reducing feelings of social isolation in at-risk parents (e.g., Home Start, van der Eyken, 1982).

Parent Has Serious Financial Difficulties

More than thirty years ago, Gil (1970) identified economic problems as a major cause for child abuse and neglect. This association has been observed many times since (e.g., Brown et al., 1998; Straus & Smith, 1990). However, it is not poverty and low income per se, but relative poverty where parents feel that they are economically disadvantaged within their community (Murray, Gakidou & Frenk, 1999; Wilkinson, 1994). This perception creates stress in the family, which then may increase the chances of aggression between family members.

The most significant problem of parents' lifestyles in the 21st century is the easy availability of loans, credit cards and store cards, whereby families can spend far beyond their means and go heavily into debt within a very short period of time. It would not be inappropriate for health professionals to enquire sensitively about the stresses caused in relation to family debt.

Parent Has Indifferent Feelings

Research for the past twenty years has demonstrated that maltreating parents have poorer quality of interaction with their infants being less reciprocal and insensitive (Browne & Saqi, 1988b; Hyman, Parr & Browne, 1979). In addition, maltreating parents have more unrealistic expectations of their child (Putallaz et al., 1998) and attribute more negative intentions to their child's behaviour in comparison to non-abusing parents (Zeanah & Zeanah, 1989). Parental attributions towards the child have also been associated with child abuse and neglect (Stratton & Swaffer, 1988). Less sensitive care-giving is claimed to dramatically impact on the infant's behaviour, increasing the chances of an insecure attachment from infant to parent and influencing the early mental representation of social relationships (Morton & Browne, 1998). Thus, abused children may develop an insensitive prototype for social relationships, as represented by their emotionally unavailable parents, who are unresponsive and rejecting. Indeed, negative attributions and behaviours of parents abused as children facilitate the intergenerational continuity of child maltreatment (Dixon, Hamilton-Giachritsis & Browne, 2005).

Interventions that promote positive parenting skills have shown some success and secure relationships between children and their parents (Sanders & Cann, 2002). Even brief interventions that include video feedback and a personal homework book have resulted in enhanced maternal sensitivity in both biological and adoptive families (see Juffer et al., 2005).

INDEX OF NEED

The Index of Need (see Table 3.3) has been developed as an assessment tool based on the above risk factors that can be used antenatally and during the infant's first year of life. It links risk factors together to provide a score that helps health and social care professionals identify families that are likely to require additional services to help them in parenting. The weighting of the factors is especially important when the risk factors occur in combination. Some combinations are much more dangerous than others and this will be indicated from the overall score.

ETHICAL CONSIDERATIONS FOR SCREENING

There are always ethical issues raised by any process of assessment. This is particularly the case when the assessment involves identifying children and families 'in need'. Therefore, the parents' understanding of the function of the assessment is crucial.

Professional practice and screening procedures for child health care and protection are legally based (Children Act, 1989, 2004; UNCRC, 1989) on the principle of what is in the best interest of the child. However, in the UK, emphasis is also placed on working in partnership with parents (Children Act, 1989, 2004), where information is shared between the parent and the health professional, and the parent takes an active role in the assessment process.

Parents must be encouraged to understand that a high number of 'risk' factors are associated with increased risk of adverse effects for the child and

Table 3.3 Index of Need

Complications during birth/separated from baby at birth because of poor health	1
You or your partner under 21 years of age	1
You or your partner are not biologically related to the child	1
Twins or less than 18 months between births of a newborn and previous children	1
You or your partner have a child with a physical or mental disability	1
You or your partner feel isolated with no one to turn to	1
You or your partner have serious financial problems	2
You or your partner have been treated for mental illness or depression	2
You or your partner feel that you have a dependency for drugs or alcohol	2
You or your partner were physically or sexually abused as a child	2
Your infant is (a) seriously ill (b) premature (c) weighed under 2.5 kgs at birth	2
You are a single parent	3
There is an adult in the house with violent tendencies	3
You or your partner are having indifferent feelings about your baby	3

A score of 5 or over indicates that a child may be 'in-need' and that a family may require referral and additional resources.

family, but that this is by no means inevitable. Parents with a high number of risk factors have a number of factors in their lives that mean they may require more support than other families. However, risk factors in themselves do not tell the whole story. It is also important to consider how the parents respond to and deal with these factors and any external sources of support they have accessed. For example, individuals will respond in very different ways to a history of childhood maltreatment, some will have sought counselling and it is important to consider how supportive or otherwise is the relationship with the child's other parent. Furthermore, a high number of risk factors places these families in high priority for support and services, which can assist in achieving a positive outcome.

Thus, it is important to highlight that this is not a punitive approach nor that a negative outcome is an inevitability, rather something that indicates they may need some extra support, which will be made available to them. It is important not to increase feelings of anxiety or stress through the parent feeling they are being negatively 'judged'. The family should not feel stigmatised in any way so it is essential that negative labels (such as 'high risk family') are discouraged in professional practice and that positive labels (such as 'family in priority') are used instead. Most importantly, a high Index of Need score placing a family in priority for services does not mean that maltreatment of the child is unavoidable. Indeed, the whole purpose of the CARE programme is the prevention of adverse outcomes for the child and family before they begin.

Therefore, the CARE programme emphasises that home visit evaluations of the child's needs and the parents' capacity to meet those needs must be carried out by the parents and health professional together. The parents are in the best position to clearly identify and indicate what social and environmental factors are affecting their capacity to care for their child's needs, but may often require reflection and support from the health professional in order to acknowledge their difficulties.

USING THE INDEX OF NEED IN THE CARE PROGRAMME

The Index of Need is not just a checklist to tick off or questions to ask. The approach of the CARE programme is to involve parents in the whole process of identifying their needs and agreeing on the best way forward of providing help and support. The 'partnership approach' is the basis for work with families with infants in the first year of life and parents remain active participants in the total process rather than as recipients of services or assessments. The aim of providing the Index of Need for parents to look at and discuss is to empower them to speak about their situation in order to mobilise the most appropriate services that will benefit them and their children. They may delay speaking about some of these issues until they feel safe and confident in the relationship with the health or social care professional.

The Index of Need is not designed to select children who are likely to suffer significant harm when it is undertaken in isolation from behavioural observations of attachment. It is designed to identify children who may be 'in need' and identify a priority service that will be required for the family to minimise or prevent the effects of the identified factors from deteriorating into serious concerns. The Index of Need also can act as a catalyst to allow those parents who just wish to talk or share a persistent problem with someone outside the family that they can trust.

WORKING IN PARTNERSHIP WITH PARENTS

One of the main principles of the Children Act (1989, 2004) is working in partnership with parents. Parents are encouraged to consider their own needs and the needs of their child, in partnership with professionals to determine what kind of support and services the family may require. On first sight, it may seem that working in partnership with parents and using the Index of Need are diametrically opposed. In fact, if the therapeutic approach is to empower the parents to talk about issues in their lives that have upset them or have created problems for them, then it does become much easier to think with them about the type of support they may require. 'Partnership with parents' is a collaborative approach to assessment and treatment that acknowledges the sharing of expertise (D'Ath & Pugh, 1986; McConkey, 1985).

The principles of working in partnership with parents have been incorporated into the CARE programme, both during assessment and the interventions that follow. In Essex, the intervention component has adopted the Parent Advisor Model of working with families in primary health care (Davis, Day & Bidmead, 2002).

Before the Children Act (1989), parents often felt that professionals did not listen to them adequately, treat them with respect or care for them as individuals with their own competencies. It is easy for professionals to consider themselves as the experts and become out of touch with how the parents are feeling, the stresses they are under and the everyday problems that they are facing. The CARE programme approach to working with parents in the community provides an excellent way of breaking down the professional-parent barrier particularly when parents are fearful of or resentful towards authority figures. It helps the community nurse think about herself in a supportive, 'enabling' role that enables the parents to function more effectively rather than as the provider of good advice.

The aims of helping identified by Hilton et al. (2002) include:

- Do no harm – professionals need to be careful that while trying to help they do not make the situation worse, precipitate further problems or increase the level of distress.
- Identify, clarify and manage problems – help parents identify and be clear about the problems they are facing.
- Facilitate the well being of children – keep in mind that all intervention should be aimed at improving the welfare of the children in the family.
- Enable parents – parents may need help to manage their own personal problems by strengthening themselves and increasing their self-confidence.
- Promote social support – parents may need help to build and strengthen social support networks with family and friends so that they are not isolated when coping with their children.
- Enable service support – providing information about local support services is essential to help parents cope.

- Predict future difficulties – parents may need help to anticipate future problems and prepare themselves to prevent problems before they arise.
- Compensate where necessary – although it is preferable to work with and through the parents there may be situations where the parents require additional support.

These points encapsulate a sensitive and responsive service to families and should be embraced by all professionals working with the parents.

Working in 'partnership' can feel threatening to some professionals who are not used to it. They may be concerned that parents will challenge their views or the accuracy of their observations. They may feel insecure with a sense of a loss of power and may feel less knowledgeable. However, each partner has something of value to contribute, power is shared and decisions are made jointly. Parents are empowered and work towards a common and explicit goal conjointly with the professionals. Therefore, the necessary elements for an effective partnership between professional and client include:

- Working together – successful outcome requires the efforts of both parents and professionals.
- Power sharing – decision-making is shared and consensus is reached whenever possible.
- Common aim – there should be an agreement to work together to pursue the same aim and have the same goals.
- Complementary expertise – parents and professionals both have differing expertise which can be combined for the desired outcome.
- Mutual respect – professionals need to earn their respect from the parents and this is often achieved by showing respect for the parents.
- Open communication – this needs to be accurate and honest.
- Negotiation – disagreements need to be managed via negotiation and attempts made to identify the source of conflict and resolve it.

The basis for partnership is trust and a good relationship. Without this communication fails and the helping process often becomes ineffective. The significant therapeutic qualities that contribute to this are genuineness, warmth and empathy (Browne, 1995; Truax & Carkhuff, 1967). 'Active listening' is an essential skill in any therapeutic relationship. It involves attending and being receptive to any information that the parents provide whether it be verbal or non-verbal. The listener poses questions to clarify what the parent has said, reflects back to the parents what they are saying in order to confirm clarification and empathy, and tries to understand the world through the eyes of the parents. The active listener has to try not to evaluate or judge what is being said but understand it first and then help the parent evaluate it once the feelings have been communicated (Egan, 1990). A sympathetic ear can be a great asset to parents who are feeling confused, frightened or stressed. Helping them organise or label their thoughts and feelings may be all that is required for them to be able to cope on their own.

Davis et al. (2002) list the fundamental professional attitudes for effective professional-client communication and outcome:

- Respect – this is an essential quality that allows the professional to value the parents as individuals and to think positively about them regardless of their problems, status, nationality, values or temperament. They need to be treated with courtesy, listened to and allowed to speak freely, even if their views are disagreed with.
- Genuineness – the professional needs to be open to experience, perceive it accurately and not distort it with their own attitudes, problems or beliefs. This implies honesty and sincerity.
- Humility – the professional needs to be realistic about what they can offer, aware of their limitations and accept the contributions of others.
- Empathy – professionals need to try to understand the world from the parent's viewpoint.
- Personal integrity – the professional needs to be relatively secure and not emotionally vulnerable in themselves so that they can cope with the distress of others.
- Quiet enthusiasm – this is important for the motivation of the profes-sional and is easily transmitted to parents and children.

If a partnership approach is utilised throughout the contact with the family, then any decision becomes a joint process where the parents are fully aware of the problems that they are trying to face and can evaluate how successful they are at coping. Take up of services should improve as parents under-stand the value of those services to themselves rather than seeing them as stigmatising or irrelevant. Professionals will be able to tailor their advice to the needs of the family they are with and parents will be able to use the help more effectively as they understand its basis and recognise how it will help.

INTRODUCING THE 'LOOKING AT YOUR NEEDS' BOOKLET

The 'Looking at your needs' booklet for midwives (see Appendix 1) and health visitors (see Appendix 2) both contain the Index of Need. This is for parents to read in advance, before discussing it with the midwife or health visitor. It is one way of giving the parents space and time to reflect on its contents, or perhaps to discuss it with each other, and raises issues in the parents' lives that they may feel unsure about whether they should mention. They may even feel that they did not know that they could talk about these kinds of issues with their health visitor. They may be surprised that these issues are of relevance to their role as parents or they may harbour secret worries that this allows them to share. It is recommended that the health professional introduce the 'Looking at your Needs' booklet in the following way:

> I've brought along this booklet for you to keep which is designed to give you information that could be useful to you and your baby. It explains how many parents feel when they first become parents or when they have another baby. There is a list of family situations written in there that may apply to you and you may wish to speak about next time we meet. It may be helpful for you to take some time to read it and think about how you want to answer the questions. When we discuss these at a later appointment we can work out which services will be most helpful to you and your family. Your answers can help me to ensure that I provide a service that meets your needs.

The aim is to help the parents speak about these issues on their own terms and in their own time if they choose to do so. If they choose not to complete the Index of Need, it is their right and choice. They may feel unsure about what is expected of them, feel that they need to keep difficult family matters to themselves or are mistrustful and wary of all professionals. It may be too early in the development of the relationship for them to trust their health visitor but they may feel able to discuss these issues once they feel more confident that they will not be misunderstood. It is important to be sensitive to the parents' reaction to the booklet and ensure that time is provided to listen to their responses. Most parents find the information helpful as it empowers them to make their own decisions. The professional needs to be aware that this is a sensitive area and they should not expect the parents to fill it in while they wait. Parents should not be pressured to complete it if they choose not to and no direct questions should be asked about the characteristics of the Index of Need. However, many comments by both parents and health professionals are positive (see Tables 3.4 and 3.5).

When parents have had the booklet for a few weeks and the health visitor or midwife returns at the four–six week visit, the subject can be raised. The aim is to empower the parents to talk about some personal issues that they may find difficult. They need an opportunity to raise issues that they may not have mentioned to anyone else, or may not have thought that they could raise with the health visitor. An empathic and understanding attitude will enable the parents to open up and share their worries.

- Have you had a chance yet to look at the booklet?
- Did you find it useful?

Table 3.4 Parents' reactions to the 'Looking at your Needs' booklet, as reported by health visitors

- The vast majority of parents are happy to complete the Index of Need.
- Parents expressed a wish to have had this information when previous babies were born.
- Many parents said that they did not realise that they could speak to health professionals about these issues.
- Parents are usually open and disclose further information on each issue.
- Parents have said it was a relief to be able to speak about unmentionable things like abuse and violence in the family.
- Parents have made very relevant remarks about wanting help to control their excessive behaviour in relation to alcohol, drugs and violence, but have never felt able to say so before.

Table 3.5 Health visitors' comments on the 'Looking at your Needs' booklet

- The information has enabled parents to speak out about their difficulties.
- Health visitors say they have been able to help parents, especially those who are adult survivors of abuse.
- The Index of Need helps health visitors prioritise services and identify children in need much sooner.
- Health visitors say that the booklet helps parents to be open and reflective.
- Health visitors feel there is less 'crisis visiting' as a result of disclosures from parents, which enables planning.

- Is there anything that you would like to discuss in there?
- What did you think of that list of factors? Did you manage to complete it? What score did you give yourself?

If the parents say 'no' and do not wish to pursue it further, which is rare, then the health visitor should accept that decision.

That's fine, no problem. Perhaps you will have time to look at it another time. I guess you've been very busy. Can I just check that I have got my information correct though?

The health visitor can then relay some general information that is already known:

- Age
- Parity
- Single/married/co-habitee
- Any other facts known, e.g., the child's illness/disability/weight at birth/prematurity

This provides an incomplete score, but this can be given to the parent and left open for discussion at a later date, if they wish to.

> That's very helpful. I have partly filled in that list in your booklet and the score is ? at the moment. Perhaps you will be able to complete that at some time if you decide it is relevant or feel able to do so.

If during this discussion the health visitor acknowledges, for example, that mother is single and living in poor accommodation or even homeless, this can lead to practical suggestions for support. This can include raising issues around how isolated she may feel while caring for her baby, any problems she is facing and whether attendance at a drop in centre or at a local group for new mothers may be helpful. Working with the mother to recognise her own needs and to enable her to accept help without feeling threatened or labelled is a very important part of facilitating access to existing services. Gentle questions or suggestions about how the mother may be feeling can be a way into the discussion.

- I wonder how you feel trying to manage on your own with your baby all of the time.
- I guess it must feel quite stressful at times or even lonely. Babies can be very demanding and can make you feel very tired.
- It can be helpful to have others to talk to about how it feels being a new mum and how to cope with noisy babies. Do you have anyone to turn to?

The aim is to work with the parents and empower them to speak about their own situation in order to mobilise appropriate services that will benefit their needs and identify children who may be high priority.

If you are concerned about the welfare or safety of the infant then the 'partnership' relationship needs to be reconsidered. Your role is primarily to act in the child's best interests, but how you do this is negotiable with the parents as long as the outcome is sound and will achieve the desired results. If, for example, a mother is only feeding her baby every six hours, refuses to feed him more than four times in 24 hours and the baby is losing weight, then the health visitor needs to raise this with the mother and point out that the baby is not receiving sufficient nutrition for healthy growth and development and that this is a direct result of the mother's strategy. The health visitor can then explore with the mother about why she feels this way and what are her reasons. The mother may be short of money or find breast feeding unpleasant. Feeds may not fit in with what she needs to do in the day or she may feel chaotic and not be able to establish a routine for the baby. The health visitor can provide support by observing feeds if the mother is finding feeding stressful, very slow or difficult.

Advice and practical help in how best to support the mother can overcome the problem but if the mother has an irrational and fixed attitude then the health visitor will need to inform her that this issue will be raised with the GP and perhaps social services. There may be concern about poor attachment, the parent may be of low intellect, or the parent may have misguided information that needs correction. The mother may feel that her baby is too greedy and that she wants a small doll-like baby that is not fat. Distorted attitudes or negative attributions about the baby need to be picked up so that the health professional can assess the level of protection the baby requires and the level of help that the mother needs.

In order for health professionals to consider distorted attitudes and negative attributions in parents, and to relate this to any concern over parental 'bonding' to the infant or infant attachment to the parent, the emotional development of infants and their parents needs to be understood.

4

THE EMOTIONAL DEVELOPMENT OF INFANTS AND THEIR PARENTS

When we think about the development of young infants, we tend to concentrate on their physical needs and their developmental needs but less commonly on their emotional needs. Any textbook about children will identify changes and growth in cognitive development, language development and intellectual development and there are well standardised tests to assess infants' developments in these areas. However, the area of emotional development is less clear and not so easily delineated. For example, what do we mean by emotional development and how does it change over time? It seems to include a mixture of features that include:

- Emotional expression – the ability to express a range of emotions, e.g., fear, anxiety, happiness, excitement, contentment, anger, frustration. The child's expression of these emotions changes with age and therefore it is difficult to describe at which age children begin to express various emotions, how they mature over time or how they learn to manage them.
- Awareness of others' feelings and emotions – empathy and sensitivity to the feelings of others link into caring and nurturing skills later in life.
- Social skills – includes the ability to be emotionally aware in contact with others, which starts with learning to share, taking turns, negotiating, managing conflicts, asserting one's needs, etc.
- Self awareness – self esteem and self confidence are part of how we value ourselves and the core sense of self that we communicate to others.
- Temperamental style – infants show a variety of different temperamental states, which link to the later development of personality.
- Level of emotional security – all the above factors are strongly associated with the emotional security of the infant. If the infant has an insecure

attachment to their parents due to the lack of parental sensitivity, consistency and availability, then all the above features of emotional development are affected.

Children's emotional development is affected and altered by their experiences with their parents and their early caretaking environment. They learn which emotions and behaviours elicit a response from their carers and their emotional expression is consequently modified.

An extreme example of this in recent years has been the behaviours and emotions shown by Romanian orphans brought up in severely emotionally deprived institutional environments. These young children's physical needs were being partially met, but their emotional needs were not being met at all. They demonstrated passive, expressionless faces, rocking and self-stimulating behaviour, and made no demands or attempts to initiate social contact. They were found to be severely delayed in their cognitive and social functioning (Kaler & Freeman, 1994). Adoption in the UK before the age of six months resulted in a dramatic catch up and recovery to within the normal range of cognitive development by four years of age as measured on the McCarthy Scales. However, this was not true of emotional development. If they were adopted after the age of six months, they still showed a marked catch up but not as great as the earlier group (Rutter et al., 1998). The research so far does not allow a distinction to be made between the effect of nutritional and psychological privation as the Romanian infants experienced both in institutional settings. However, when the children's social and emotional development were examined, there was a close association between the duration of the children's deprivation and the severity of their attachment disorder (O'Connor et al., 1999, 2000, 2003).

Hence, the child's social and emotional experiences in the first year of life are critical for later development. Children who are placed in residential care rather than family-based care (e.g., foster care) are at risk of harm due to the institutional nature of their environment (Browne et al., 2005). There is also growing clinical evidence that later adoption of children in mid-childhood who have suffered severe neglect or abuse in their early years does not repair the early emotional damage. They continue to have major relationship and behavioural difficulties. Therefore, intervention with children who are emotionally at risk within their families needs to be very early, immediate and effective in order to prevent the later continuation of problems. Indeed, over 30 years ago, Clarke and Clarke (1976) commented that children in adversity require a permanent placement before the age of three years to avoid any later developmental problems.

Table 4.1 Essential needs of children that must be satisfied by 'good-enough' parenting

Physical needs	Behavioural needs	Emotional needs
Nutrition	Stimulation/interaction	Affection/empathy
Warmth/shelter	Exploration/learning	Availability
Health/cleanliness	Socialisation/role model	Consistency/routine
Safety	Limit setting	Sensitivity
Protection	Rest/sleep	Attachment/autonomy
Contact/comfort	Play	Individual identity
Immunisation		Building of self esteem
		Advocacy

Adapted from Reder & Lucey, 1995.

'GOOD ENOUGH' PARENTING

The basic needs of children are reflected in attempts to define 'good enough' parenting, a term coined by Winnicot (1960). This term indicates the parent's ability to recognise and respond to the child's needs without having to be a perfect parent all of the time. 'Good enough' parents facilitate age appropriate development within a safe environment (Adcock & White, 1985, 1998). Every child has a need for:

- basic physical care, security and safety
- affection and approval
- discipline and control that are consistent and age appropriate
- teaching and stimulation
- provision of normal life experiences
- encouragement of appropriate levels of independence
- response to changing needs and awareness that the needs have precedence over the parent's needs
- positive role models (Parameswaran, 1997).

Table 4.1 delineates what is considered essential in parenting. As previously described in the Framework for Assessment of Children and their Families (Dept of Health et al., 2000), the parents are assessed on the basis of their capacity to meet the needs of the child, taking into account any social and environmental factors that might affect that capacity.

THE PRENATAL PARENT-INFANT RELATIONSHIP

Attachment between the mother and her infant starts prenatally. Daniel Stern (1995, 1998) has been an influential theorist in the area of understanding the complexity of parent-infant relationships. He describes the 'represented' baby as having a long prenatal history (Stern, 1995). As the foetus grows and develops, there is a parallel development in the mother's mind. At around four months of gestation, there is a leap in the richness and specificity of the mother's 'representations' of her foetus-as-an-infant, partly triggered by the ultra sound examination that is often done at this time. It is also the time when she starts to feel the foetus move and the prospective baby seems more real. Between the fourth and seventh month of gestation there is a rapid growth in the richness, quantity and specificity of the thoughts about the baby. From seven months, most parents are more preoccupied with preparing themselves for the birth of the child. Sometimes parents may contemplate and fear that their hopes and expectations may not be met, but this is balanced by the excitement of giving birth. Indeed, most mothers report that the pain of labour and delivery is quickly forgotten following the birth of the child.

It is claimed that mothers' descriptions of their babies before birth can be used to predict the level of infant security of attachment after birth (Benoit et al., 1997; Fonagy et al., 1991; Ward & Carlson, 1995). There does appear to be a concordance between the mothers' description of their babies and the infant attachment to the parent, as well as stability in the parent's perceptions during pregnancy and throughout the first year of life (Mebert, 1989, 1991; Zeanah et al., 1985, 1987).

However, many prenatal classes for parents emphasise the medical perspective of pregnancy and focus on childbirth rather than exploring or assisting emotional adjustment to parenthood (Combes & Schonveld, 1993). Often, it is parents' recollections and feelings about their own experiences of being parented as a child that are critical in the development of their own parenting skills and how they feel about themselves (Fonagy, 1998). Parents who are supported in pregnancy are psychologically healthier, suffer less anxiety and depression, and experience more satisfaction in their relationships with their baby and their partner (Fonagy, 1998). This indicates that work with the mother prior to birth can be an important period for identifying future possible difficulties in attachment and in coping with being a parent.

THE PARENT-INFANT RELATIONSHIP

It is widely recognised that an infant's first relationship with their primary care-giver is the most important relationship of their lives and is the basis for how the person socially interacts and develops other emotional relationships – the internal working model (Bowlby, 1969). The primary care-giver is not necessarily the biological mother, it could be any male or female adult who provides care. However, on most occasions, the biological mother is the primary focus of the infant's first relationship.

Many researchers of mother-infant interaction and infant development have emphasised that the mother provides an emotional and behavioural structure or 'scaffold' on which the infant builds their social and mental experiences (Schaffer, 1977, 1990; Whiten, 1977). Siblings and other adults, such as fathers, can also be important sources of interaction and developmental influence (Dunn, 1993; Dunn & Kendrick, 1982).

Stern (1995) describes the mother-infant interaction where the mother, father and infant interact with each other (see Figure 4.1, central circles), but how they interact is determined to a degree by their internal 'representations' of each other. These 'representations' include their memories of previous interactions and personal interpretations of the interaction.

Stern describes family interaction as being interpreted and perceived through different lenses particular to each person in the interaction: '*There are lenses of fantasies, hopes, fears, family traditions and myths, important personal experiences, current pressures and many other factors*' (Stern, 1998, p. 12). He sees the parent-infant relationship as existing in two parallel worlds:

- The real, objectifiable external world, i.e., the real baby in the real mother's arms.
- The imaginary, subjective, mental world of representations, i.e., the imagined baby in the arms of the imagined self-as-mother.

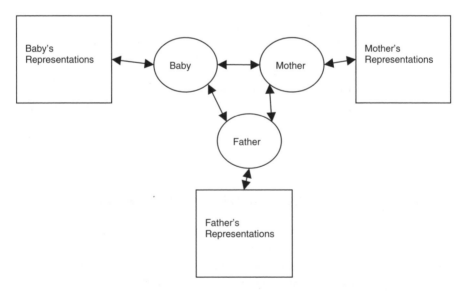

Figure 4.1 Stern's model of relationship development in families (1995)

Stern (1995) developed his analysis of the early infant-mother relationship to include a construct that he calls the 'motherhood constellation'. He sees this period as unique, dominant, variable in length and entirely normal. Once the baby is born the mother has several new questions and anxieties in her life that dominate how she thinks, feels and behaves:

- Can I keep my baby alive?
- Can I love my baby?
- Who will help and look after me while I look after my baby?
- Will I be a good mother?

Stern's psychodynamic ideas and the above construct have been the basis for therapeutic work and prevention with expectant and new parents to enhance the quality of their relationships with their baby, e.g., PIPPIN (Parents in Partnership-Parents Infant Network; Parr, 1998).

Stern (1995) has identified a number of clinical windows through which the early parent-infant relationship can be viewed:

- 0–2.5 months. The major interactive tasks are around regulation of the baby's feeding, sleep/wake and activity cycles and the majority of interchanges take place around these events. Observation of these events can provide considerable insight into the ability of the mother to be sensitive and responsive to her baby, their temperamental fit, the level of control or bizarreness.
- 2.6–5.5 months. Observation of face-to-face social interaction without toys or other objects between mother and infant shows the mutual regulation of the social interchange. The baby is able to control gaze, responsive smiling and vocalising by this age and both parent and infant have equal control, contributing to the initiation, maintenance, modulation, termination or avoidance of the face-to-face play.
- 5.6–8 months. Observation of joint object play can demonstrate the direction, timing, focus, change of object and disengagement of play. For example, the level of maternal intrusiveness and over-control can provide a clear indication of her inability to recognise her baby's contribution to the interaction.
- 9–12 months. The pattern of infant attachment to the parent is usually very clear by this age and observing how the parent and infant negotiate separation and return can provide valuable insight into the security of the attachment. Separation and reunion have been the standard behaviour for assessing attachment but, equally, showing affection, seeking comfort, reliance for help and cooperation are important indicators (Zeanah et al., 1993).

The development of person/object permanence and inter-subjectivity are evident from 9–12 months. The infant is able to realise that the mother is a separate person and has a separate mind from his or her own. It is possible to observe social referencing, affect attunement, joint attention getting and reading of each other's intentions. In addition, children will readily retrieve hidden objects after searching for them.

At each stage of development, the infant assimilates new experiences in the social and physical environment and then accommodates these new experiences into his or her cognitions and behaviours (Piaget, 1954). Hence, the infant builds on previous experiences to develop a repertoire of skilled actions and reactions. It is possible to observe the parent and infant negotiating these newly found skills at each stage of infant development, which are mainly sensorimotor and representational in nature (Bruner et al., 1956; Piaget, 1954).

Parental Bonding to the Infant

The transition to parenthood is a critical period in human development and requires social and emotional support from others. With the birth come enormous changes in the mother's basic status and identity, some of which will have been anticipated but others will be unforeseen. One important change is the transition from being a daughter-of-her-mother to being a mother-of-her-daughter/son (Stern, 1995). This irreversible shift in perspective produces many of the positive and negative fantasies, hopes and fears of new mothers (e.g., 'I will never behave the way my mother did to me'; 'I want to be just like my mother'). The new mother starts to re-evaluate her relationship with her own mother. There appears to be a strong intergenerational influence in parenting and the nature of the mother's current representation of her own mother as a parent may be an important influence on the pattern of attachment that the mother will establish with her infant by 12 months of age (Zeanah & Barton, 1989). For example, the Adult Attachment Interview (AAI) for assessing parental childhood attachment memories (Main, Kaplan & Cassidy, 1985), has been administered prenatally to mothers. The responses to the AAI predicted infants' attachment classification on the Strange Situation Test one year later with 81% accuracy (Benoit & Parker, 1994).

There is also another significant mental shift in the mother, where she should begin to put the baby's interests and needs before her own. Some mothers find this particularly difficult to do and this may reflect on their own unmet parenting needs as a child. Their emotional immaturity will significantly affect their ability to parent well.

Zeanah et al. (1994) have developed a 'Working Model of the Child Interview' (WMCI) to investigate the care-giver's perceptions and subjective experience of their infant's individual characteristics and their relationship with their child. This one hour structured interview categorises responses of the parent into different features:

- Content features that include how difficult the infant is perceived to be and how much fear for the infant's safety is expressed by the parents.
- Affective tone includes the parent's expressed joy, pride, anger, disappointment, anxiety, guilt, indifference and other emotions.
- Qualitative scales include the richness of the perceptions, openness to change, intensity of involvement, coherence, caregiving, sensitivity and acceptance.

Parents' perceptions of the infant are classified as balanced, disengaged or distorted (see Table 4.2).

Benoit et al. (1997) looked at whether the mothers' narrative descriptions of their infants as measured on the WMCI were related to their infants' attachment classification on the Strange Situation Test (Ainsworth et al., 1978) and found that they were concordant on the positive relationships, i.e., a balanced maternal representation was correlated with a securely attached infant. However, they did not find concordance between a disengaged representation and an avoidant attachment or a distorted representation and a resistant attachment. They also found that the mothers' representations of their infants as assessed by the WMCI remain stable and can predict infants' attachment one year later with 74% accuracy. What is important is that the narrative features of a mother's descriptions of her infant can predict infant security of attachment after birth.

The parent's beliefs about the causes of the infant's behaviour can affect their reactions to the infant (Crittenden, 2002). For example, abusing mothers have been found to attribute more control and more internal causes to the infant than to themselves compared to non-abusing mothers or mothers of handicapped children (Stratton & Swaffer, 1988). Comments about the infant deliberately making a noise, being attention seeking at night, or never satisfied with a feed can be indicators of negative attributions. The parent may even give the impression of the baby being malicious in intent or deliberately interfering with the parent's life.

In relation to the CARE programme and the Index of Need, families with a high number of risk factors are considered to be in need of further support and services in order to prevent the possibility of child abuse and neglect. However, research has shown (Browne & Saqi, 1987) that families in priority ('high risk' families) differ from families who are already maltreating their children by the fact that they have more positive views of their infant's behaviour. These positive perceptions and attributions act as a buffer against stressful risk factors reducing the likelihood of harm to the child and enhance

Table 4.2 Classifications of parental perceptions of their infant using the 'Working Model of the Child Interview'

Classification	Features
Balanced ('mostly realistic')	Includes both positive and negative characteristics of the infant or the care-giver's relationship with the infant. The parent recognises and values the baby's individuality, they are engrossed in the relationship and empathically appreciate the baby's own experiences. The parent is open to change, can take in new information about the baby and parenting instead of being rigid and inflexible.
Disengaged ('occasionally realistic')	The parent describes the baby in cool tones, with emotional distance or indifference. The baby's own world seems strange to the parent who does not seem to know the baby as an individual. There may be an absence of genuine interest or curiosity about the baby. Details about the baby and parenting are poor and limited in quality and there is inflexibility about taking in new information. The parents dismiss the importance of the impact of their relationship with the baby and that it will have an effect on the baby's development.
Distorted ('rarely realistic')	The parent may have unrealistic expectations, attribute deliberate intent to the baby or is insensitive to the baby as an individual. These parents may expect the baby to please them or be excessively compliant. They fail to recognise the impact of their parenting on the baby. If they are overwhelmed or preoccupied by other concerns they may seem confused or overwhelmed by the baby's demands. Their description of the baby may seem incoherent, i.e. confused, contradictory or even bizarre. Strong feelings may be expressed but they lack control or contextual meaning.

Adapted from Zeanah et al., 1994.

the possibility of sensitive parent-child interaction (Browne & Herbert, 1997).

In the Browne and Saqi (1987) study of 16 maltreating, 35 'high risk' and 39 'low risk' parents responses to a child behaviour checklist (Richman, Stevenson & Graham, 1982), it was shown that maltreating mothers were significantly more likely to negatively rate their children's feeding and sleeping patterns and claim they were miserable and irritable in comparison to 'high' and 'low' risk mothers. However, direct observations of the children by the researchers in their homes showed no significant differences between the children across the three groups (see Table 4.3). These differences between maltreating and high risk parents' perceptions and attributions are despite the fact that they have similar levels of life stress events (see Table 4.4).

In addition, the maltreating and high risk mothers also showed higher levels of postnatal depression (63.6% and 47.9% respectively) during the first 12 months post-delivery compared to low risk mothers (32%). Therefore, it can be asserted that parents' positive perceptions and attributions of the child protect the relationship in the presence of stressful events and situations, and may even help the parent maintain positive interactions when they are depressed.

Postnatal Depression and its Effect on Infant-mother Attachment

Maternal depression is generally associated with a higher incidence of behavioural problems and psychopathology in children (Gelfand & Teti, 1990), and postnatal depression has been associated with delayed cognitive

Table 4.3 Frequency of low, medium and high child behaviour checklist scores from 'low risk', 'high risk' and maltreating parents

	'Low risk' (N = 39)		'High risk' (N = 35)		Maltreating (N = 16)	
	n	%	n	%	n	%
Low score (0–7)	25	64.1	14	40.0	5	31.3
Medium score (8–14)	14	35.9	20	57.1	7	43.8
High score (15–28)	0	0.0	1	2.9	4	25.0

Adapted from Browne & Saqi, 1987*.
* $\chi = 18.79$, df = 2, p < 0.001.

Table 4.4 Number of life stress events for mothers from 'low risk', 'high risk' and maltreating families during the first 12 months following delivery

	'Low risk'		'High risk'		Maltreating	
	n	%	n	%	n	%
0–3 stress factors	26	68.4	12	35.3	2	16.7
4–22 stress factors	12	31.6	22	64.7	10	83.3

Adapted from Browne & Saqi, 1987*.
* $\chi = 13.17$, df = 2, significant at p < 0.001.

development and insecure attachment in later infancy and early childhood, particularly when the infant is a boy (Murray & Cooper, 1996).

A meta-analytic study of six other studies has shown that infants of depressed mothers were less likely to show secure attachment and more likely to show avoidant or disorganised forms of attachment (Martins & Gaffan, 2000). However, these effects are not statistically strong and show variability. It appears that other influences (i.e., poverty, maltreatment, drug abuse, maternal hostility and neurological abnormalities in the child) are much stronger predictors of disorganised attachment than postnatal depression. Indeed, many factors moderate the development of the mother-infant relationship and attachment, such as infant characteristics, marital relations and social support (Belsky & Isabella, 1988).

Insensitive early interaction with the mother is associated with insecure attachment (De Wolff & van Ijzendoorn, 1987) but not with disorganised attachment (Main & Solomon, 1990). It has been proposed that mothers who experience unresolved loss or trauma were more likely to have disorganised infants with the mediating process being the mother's frightened or frightening behaviour (Schuengel et al., 1999).

Nevertheless, these findings indicate that detecting postnatal depression during home visiting after birth is a necessary and important part of the health visitor service to families with infants, because depression may have a long-term effect on infant attachment.

Attachment of the Infant to the Parent

One of the main theorists of early emotional development has been John Bowlby (1969, 1973, 1980) who described three phases in the development of infant attachment to their parent during the first year of life:

1. 0–4 months – the infant orientates to signals without differentiating between different people.
2. 5–7 months – the infant shows preferential orientation to a parent or regular carer by being more likely to smile at them or to be comforted more easily by them if distressed.
3. 7–9 months – the infant maintains proximity preferentially to parents or carers by moving towards them or crying and protesting if the person leaves.

The development of the emotional attachment between infants and parents/ carers is a critical feature of the first year of life. Babies need care and protection and indicate this by crying when they feel uncomfortable, stressed, bored or tired.

Thus, attachment behaviour is defined as proximity seeking behaviour by an infant or child when they experience any sense of discomfort including pain, fear, cold or hunger. This 'instinctive' behaviour has a biological basis as the baby is totally dependent on carer attention for their survival. The infant seeks the closeness of the parent or carer in the hope that they will reduce their discomfort and restore their equanimity (Bowlby, 1969). Babies also develop representational models, which are internal working models of relationships through the process of attachment (Bowlby, 1980). These models are dynamic representations that are based on real interactive experiences, tend to be stable over time and guide behaviour and the formation of later emotional relationships. Attachment behaviours in the baby are not just a way of maintaining proximity with the care-giver but essentially create the conditions for the development of a representation system for mental states (Fonagy, 1998). The baby gradually develops a way of interpreting its experiences in terms of a set of stable and generalised intentional attributes, i.e., desires, emotions, intentions and beliefs. The baby can then use this representation system to predict others' or their own behaviour in varying situations. This capacity to interpret behaviour and make sense of what happens is a mechanism for processing new experiences. The contingent responding of the parent or carer is the main method by which the baby tests and learns about their own internal states and then learns about the feelings and behaviours of others.

Bowlby (1988) has argued that infants develop an internal working model of themselves and their parents based on the reactions of the parents to their normal and every day demands for attention and care. These models are the beliefs that the child holds about themselves and predictions about how they will be treated by others based on their past experience. Secure attachment is necessary for the development of a secure sense of self and intermediate to high self-esteem. This enhances resilience to stress and effectively inhibits natural antisocial tendencies (Fonagy, 1998).

Babies can make multiple attachments to different adults in their lives depending on their care arrangements. Generally, attachments are made to responsive carers who interact and play a lot with the infant, but simple care-taking activities like changing nappies do not seem to be so important (Schaffer & Emerson, 1964). Often, a hierarchy of attachment figures can be identified where the baby shows a preference for one carer over another if both carers are present. This may be task related, e.g., mother when the baby is tired, hungry or unwell and father for constructive or boisterous play. This would demonstrate that the mother is the primary attachment figure and the father the secondary attachment figure.

The baby's style of attachment to the parents/carers has been measured by observing the baby's reaction to brief separation from the parent and how they behave on reunion with the parent in the Strange Situation Test

(Ainsworth et al., 1978). This test consists of a series of three minute episodes designed to elicit attachment behaviours in the laboratory setting in 12–18 month old infants. The attachment classification is based on a study of the organisation of the infant behaviour directed towards the primary caregiver during the procedure. The reliability and validity of this procedure has been well documented and it has been used in numerous studies on infant attachment (Bretherton & Waters, 1985; Cassidy & Shaver, 1999; Morton & Browne, 1998).

The psychological research findings from the Strange Situation Test have identified four categories of infant attachment:

- Type A – Anxious/avoidant attachment: these babies show conspicuous avoidance of the mother, ignore her on return and do not seek to be close to her or interact with her. During the separation the baby is not distressed and any distress is due to being left alone rather than to mother's absence.
- Type B – Secure attachment: these babies actively seek and maintain proximity, contact or interaction with the mother particularly on reunion. They may or may not be distressed during the separation but any distress is related to the mother's absence.
- Type C – Anxious/resistant attachment: these babies are usually distressed on separation but resist contact and interaction with the mother on reunion. They seek proximity but appear ambivalent about approaching the mother and may show approach/withdrawal behaviour.
- Type D – Disorganised attachment (Main & Solomon, 1990): these babies show disorganised and disoriented behaviour.

These different types of attachments have been linked to parenting experiences that the infant has been exposed to during their first year of life. There is large over-representation of the type D disorganised attachment in 12-month-old infants who have been maltreated (82%) in comparison to a non-maltreated group (19%; Carlson et al., 1989). It has been suggested that fear in the caregiving relationship leads to disorganised attachment (Main & Hesse, 1990). The frightened or discomforted infant who seeks his or her attachment figure (who is at the same time the source of his or her discomfort) will experience significant stress and ambivalence.

A review of 13 studies of infant attachment patterns in strange situations (Morton & Browne, 1998) reported an average of 76% of infants showing insecure attachments to mothers from maltreating families. This compared to 34% of infants insecurely attached to non-maltreating mothers. From the opposite perspective, this shows that 24% of maltreated infants are categorised as securely attached (compared to 66% of non-maltreated infants), despite their harmful experiences. Nevertheless, some authors claim that at

Table 4.5 Attachment patterns derived from brief separation and reunion of infant and mother in the home environment

	Ainsworth category	Abused infants (n = 23) %	'High risk' (n = 42) %	'Lower risk' (n = 46) %
Avoidant	A_1A_2	52.0	21.5	17.0
Independent	B_1B_2	9.0	50.0	48.0
Dependent	B_3B_4	9.0	19.0	24.0
Ambivalent	C_1C_2	30.0	9.5	11.0
Total number of insecure attachments		82%	31%	28%

From Hamilton & Browne, 2002.

least some of this 24% are 'falsely' categorised and may have a disorganised 'D' pattern of attachment (Carlson, Cicchetti, Barnett & Braunwald, 1989; Solomon & George, 1999). However, there have been relatively few studies of infant attachment patterns and their pathology that were carried out in the home environment compared to strange situations in clinical settings. Home-based studies are useful to community nurses in providing reliable and valid information on infant attachment patterns to their primary care-givers at home. Hamilton and Browne (2002) report an unpublished UK study of brief separation and reunion of infant and mother in the home (see Table 4.5). Abused infants again showed the highest number of insecure attachments (82%) in comparison to 'high risk' infants (31%) and 'low risk' infants (28%), as determined by the Index of Need.

Insecure infant attachment to the primary care-giver is sometimes associated with emotional abuse and neglect, which may cause significant harm to child health and development, such as failure to thrive (Iwaniec, 2004).

THE CONCEPT OF EMOTIONAL CHILD MALTREATMENT AND 'SIGNIFICANT HARM'

Predicting possible emotional abuse or neglect of the infant is a remarkably difficult decision making process (Iwaniec, 1995). Although the focus of assessment is the relationship between the baby and carer, this relationship is based within a family which is in turn influenced by the social and cultural environment to which the family belongs (Fortin & Chamberland,

1995). The development of a positive or potentially emotionally abusive relationship between the parents and the infant occurs over time and so repeated observations of the relationship can provide a valuable insight into how the infant and parents are progressing. Emotional abuse and neglect is identified when maltreatment of the infant occurs pervasively and characterises the relationship (e.g., consistent verbal abuse or the infant witnesses conflict between mother and father). The interactions are actually or potentially harmful emotionally and include omissions as well as commissions (Glaser & Prior, 2002). The definition of abuse includes qualitative as well as quantitative aspects. There can be single events, repeated events or a pattern of interaction that is characteristic of an abusive relationship. Physical or sexual abuse tends to be events but neglect and emotional abuse characterise the relationship (Glaser, 2000; Iwaniec, 1995).

The concept of 'significant harm' (Adcock & White, 1998) as defined in the Children Act (1989) has been accepted as the threshold for recognition of child abuse and neglect. Significant harm relies on evidence of either:

- ill treatment of a child that has caused or is likely to cause significant harm to the child and/or
- impairment of the child's health and development which is attributable to ill treatment or the care that the child has or has not received.

When considering the possibility of emotional abuse the health visitor needs to keep in mind the concept of 'significant harm' to activate child protection procedures. It distinguishes between ill treatment (omission and commission) by the abuser and impairment of the child's health and development (the damage sustained by the child). There is no requirement to prove the parent's or the abuser's intent to harm the child in order to satisfy the threshold (Glaser & Prior, 2002). The categories of ill treatment include:

1. **Emotional unavailability, unresponsiveness and neglect.** Parents are usually preoccupied with their own problems, i.e., mental ill health and substance abuse, and are unable rather than unwilling to respond to the baby's emotional needs.
2. **Negative attributions and misattributions to the child.** Parents show hostility towards and denigration or rejection of the baby who is seen as deserving this treatment.
3. **Developmentally inappropriate or inconsistent interaction with the child.** This includes expectations of the baby beyond his or her developmental capabilities; over protection and limitation of exploration and learning; exposure to confusing or traumatic events and interactions.
4. **Failure to recognise or acknowledge the child's individuality and psychological boundary.** Parents use the baby to fulfil the parents' own

psychological needs, or they show an inability to distinguish between the baby's reality and the adult's belief and wishes.

5. **Failing to promote the child's social adaptation.** This includes psychological neglect and failure to provide adequate cognitive stimulation or opportunities for experiential learning, or promoting mis-socialisation, e.g., corrupting.

Parents or carers need to be 'good enough' in their care to manage any infant no matter how disabled, ill, handicapped or temperamentally difficult they are. If they are having problems coping, they need to be aware enough to ask for and seek out support and help in their child care. Appropriate community based interventions will help prevent child abuse and neglect both in this generation and the next (Buchanan, 1996).

5

OBSERVATION OF PARENT-INFANT INTERACTION

In order to assess parent-infant interaction and indicators of attachment formation, it is essential to observe parents and their babies together over several sessions and to try to evaluate what is observed. The importance of observations of parent-child interaction in the home environment is that they can provide information on the quality of the relationship in terms of affection and security. A parent-child relationship is characterised by diverse interactions that vary in content and context. It is further characterised by the following parental behaviour that relates to the formation of infant attachment to the parent (Herbert, 1991; Maccoby, 1980):

- Sensitivity/reciprocity – the sensitive parent is in attunement with the infant's behaviour. He or she understands and empathises with the infant, responding consistently and appropriately, meshing his/her responses to the infant's gestures and communications to form a cyclic turn-taking pattern of interaction. This smooth reciprocal interactive pattern can be so fast as to appear simultaneous. In contrast, the insensitive parent intervenes arbitrarily and these non-reciprocal intrusions reflect his or her own wishes and mood.
- Acceptance/rejection – the accepting parent accepts and is committed to the responsibility of childcare. He or she shows few signs of irritation with the infant. However, the rejecting parent has feelings of anger and resentment that eclipse his or her affection for the infant. He or she often finds the infant irritating and resorts to punitive control.
- Co-operation/interference – the co-operative parent respects the infant's autonomy and rarely exerts direct control, but guides the infant offering a variety of experiences. The interfering parent imposes her wishes on the child with little concern for the infant's current mood or activity.
- Accessibility/ignoring – the accessible parent is familiar with his or her infant's communications and notices them at some distance, hence he or

she is easily distracted by the infant and often shows love and affection. The ignoring parent is preoccupied with his or her own activities and thoughts, and shows affection in response to their own needs. He or she often fails to notice the child's communications unless they are obvious through intensification. He or she may even forget about the infant outside the scheduled times for caretaking.

Affectionate parent-infant relationships can also be identified by the fact that the presence of the other alleviates anxiety induced by strange objects, persons or situations. The parent's actions will be conducive to the welfare of the infant and there will be an uninhibited display of affection and love. Often the parent changes and softens his or her voice when speaking to and comforting the infant. The list of questions in Table 5.1 will aid you in observing the interaction between the primary care-giver and the infant.

The community nurse is at the front line of being able to observe the interaction between parents and their infant. However, a structure and understanding of what to observe rather than basing recommendations on hunches and feelings are vital for the safety of the infants. The CARE Programme provides a plan of observation that supplements the information gained from the Index of Need and is in two main sections:

1. The parents' reactions to the infant.
2. The infant's reactions to the parents.

Table 5.1 Questions that identify a positive parent-infant relationship

Infants – do they?	Care-givers – do they?
• Appear alert	• Respond to the infant's demands
• Appear easily comforted	• Show interest in face-to-face contact with the infant
• Exhibit tolerance	• Show an ability to comfort
• Vocalise appropriately	• Identify positive and negative qualities in equal proportions
• Explore the environment	• Show pleasure at being with the infant
• Respond to care-giver(s)	• Play with the infant
• React to pain and pleasure	• Respond to the infant's messages
• Express frustration	• Praise the infant
• Respond to limit setting	• Show interest in the infant's development
• Exhibit observable fears	• Accept the expression of attempts at autonomy and independence by the infant

I. The Parents' Reaction to the Infant and Parenthood

Being aware of a parent's feelings towards his or her baby is the basis for a preventative approach to parenting problems. Listening to what the parents say about their new infant reveals many of their underlying views and assumptions. Parents need to feel able to express negative as well as positive views about their baby and how they are coping without this being judged or corrected. The stress of coping with a new life and all of the new responsibilities are overwhelming at times. Their moods will shift and depend on recent events and strains as well as how much sleep they have managed to snatch. Facilitating a discussion of how the parents feel and encouraging them to talk openly creates a more trusting relationship with the community nurse and makes the process of thinking about their needs much easier. Helping parents label their feelings, before they start labelling their children and start punishing them, can help them recognise the cause of the problems.

The aim of the CARE programme is to try to understand how the parents are feeling about parenthood and their baby. This process of assessment can start during the pregnancy when the midwife is making a relationship with the prospective mother and is able to talk to her about how she feels about being pregnant, her hopes and aspirations and how realistic she is about the future. A mother whose baby is a result of a one-night relationship may have very different feelings to one who has tried for several years to get pregnant. In one family, the imminent birth may be welcomed but is an additional stress in an already overburdened family while, in another family, the baby may have been totally unexpected and the news of the pregnancy may be treated with disbelief and horror. Helping parents through their worries, expectations and concerns during pregnancy can be a journey of possible acceptance or developing rejection. Working through anxieties, possible scenarios, problem-solving options and helping parents make decisions is all part of supporting parents during pregnancy.

Once the baby arrives, a new set of experiences, feelings and emotions develop which may or may not exacerbate the worries that preceded the birth. Supporting parents during the first few months of the baby's life is often a critical time of adjustment and including fathers is important.

One father, whose third baby had just been born, was included for the first time in discussions about the Index of Need and was really pleased that someone had bothered to ask if he had been abused as a child. It was the first time he had spoken about it to anyone. His wife had been complaining that he was not helping out with the new baby. He commented 'If only I had known about this before. I know what happened to me has affected me as a father; I've been terrified even to bathe my children and did not know what to do or how to help in their care. I've stayed away from them because I've been scared. I want this to change with this baby. I need help to be more confident in handling him and knowing that I can be a good father.' The

> parents were able to talk honestly to each other about how they felt for the first time.
>
> Another young father commented that the 'ambivalent feelings' question applied to him. He admitted that he was punitive and erratic in his feelings for the baby, and realised that he needed some help in coping and adapting to parenthood.

Midwives and health visitors need efficient and effective liaison to enable the continuity of care after birth. The information that is gained by the midwife prior to birth can be invaluable to the health visitor during the first few weeks after birth.

> One new mother seemed nervous and anxious during the health visitor's first home visit. The health visitor decided to visit the following week to weigh the baby and found the baby in the crib and the mother showing no sensitivity to the baby as she undressed him for weighing. She started to ask the mother 'What is it like being a new mother?', which immediately unleashed a torrent of distress 'It's horrible, it's dreadful. I hate it all.' The health visitor gently prompted, 'Shall we talk about why you feel like this?'. The mother burst into tears and said that she felt guilty about feeling the way she did and could not tell her partner how bad she felt because he adored the baby. She revealed that she had a history of depression, problems with relationships and had self harmed in the past.
>
> The health visitor linked her to her GP, she received antidepressants and some continued supportive visits from the health visitor. By 8 months after the birth, the mother was more open and felt that she could manage. There were no concerns that she would harm the baby and the father had been engaged in supporting her. Her feelings were acknowledged and normalised.

a) Attributions

The attributions that the parents make about the infant either before or after birth are an important indicator of the parents' feelings about the baby. A parent who is always complaining about their baby's crying, their need for feeding and changing, the lack of sleep, the strain on the finances, the baby's temper, or the continual hard work that caring for a baby creates, may be showing signs of exhaustion, incipient postnatal depression or poor attachment of the parent to the baby. The mother may be blaming or scapegoating the baby for all of the bad feelings she has, some of which may have nothing to do with the baby.

> 'I never realised how tired I would feel. He seems to be crying all the time and I never seem to have any time to do anything. I get so exhausted that I cry everyday. I feel so sad; it was all supposed to be so lovely.'
>
> 'He's a real pain. If he's not hungry he needs changing, if he's not being carried he cries. There's non-stop washing and I have no time to myself.'

'I get so worried about whether she's having enough milk. I don't know how to judge when she's full. She seems ever so greedy. She seems to want to feed every hour and I'm sure that can't be right.'

The health visitor may hear that the mother is complaining a lot about the baby but may observe a clean and well-fed baby who has a stimulating and safe environment and whose needs are understood and are being met. What the health visitor sees and hears need to be balanced. The tone of the mother's voice and non-verbal signals are important indicators. The complaints of a mother like this can be responded to with empathy and queries about what would make her feel better. Helping her recognise that she is doing a good job, that she is a good mother and pointing out her strengths can help turn the tables on how she is feeling. She needs positive feedback and appreciation, and the community nurse may be the only person who can offer her this.

Mother: He always seems to be fretting about something. I have no peace in the day. He just cries and even when I pick him up he carries on and it is so loud in my ear. I don't know what to do with him he just seems grumpy all the time and nothing I do helps.

Health visitor: It sounds as if you are feeling a bit overwhelmed by him. He's making you feel not very good about yourself and doubting your ability as a mother. It seems hard to find anything positive to say about him at the moment.

Mother: Yes, I feel absolutely helpless and find I'm really starting to dislike him. I dread waking up in the morning. My life seems to have disappeared and all I do is live with a screaming, puking baby.

Health visitor: What do you feel would help you when you are feeling so down? What would perk you up and make life look rosier?

Mother: Well, I would really love to have a long hot bath with lots of bubbles in it. Do you think it would be terrible if I left him in his cot to cry and just shut the door while I did that?

Recognising and accepting the mother's feelings about her baby is the first step in being able to help improve the situation. Some preventative work at this stage can be helpful in controlling the escalating distress of the mother and help her take a more balanced look at her life and her baby. The health visitor has a repertoire of skills that she brings to the relationship with the parent, which can help the mother. She can:

- focus on some of the positive elements of the baby
- think of options to solve the problem

- consider options for support from partner, family, friends or support groups
- think of ways of getting her own life back on course
- learn how to cope with the stresses of baby's crying and sleeping
- think of treats for herself to feel human again
- check out any worries she has about the health of the baby.

An assessment of the safety of the baby is critical in the early weeks and months of life. It is important to remember that even when a baby is ill (e.g., has gastro-oesophageal reflux and is crying, vomiting and refusing to feed) that a parent will still be able to demonstrate love and affection, sympathy and concern. However, a parent who feels that their baby is crying deliberately to upset them is of much more concern.

Parents will often try to find similarities in their baby's looks, temperament and behaviour to themselves or to relatives, with bad features often being compared to disliked family members. Some mothers fear that their baby will show the bad characteristics of themselves or the other parent. If the father is no longer around, there may be worries about what the baby will be like, with temper and aggression being the major concerns. They will group features together or may be able to select both positive and negative features.

- cuddly/loving/smiley/giggly/feeds well/sleeps well/contented
- whinging/irritable/never satisfied/demanding/hungry/tired/angry
- unpredictable/unsettled/startles/wriggly
- detached/unresponsive/serious/watchful/uncuddly.

> 'She's got such a bad temper, just like her dad, and she's a red head too, just like him, but she has such a great smile.'
>
> 'He wriggled non-stop inside me and now he hasn't stopped since he came out. The nurse in the hospital said I had a right one here and he was going to cause me a lot of grief. Do you think it's a sign that he's going to be very clever?'
>
> 'He seems not to want to be cuddled, he wriggles when I pick him up and starts to cry so I put him down and leave him alone. He isn't anything like I thought he would be and I don't understand him.'

An assessment is made of the parents' attributions at each visit in the first year of life and this will provide a picture of whether the parents change these attributions as the baby grows older (see Table 5.2). A continual pattern of negative attribution needs to be viewed in the context of the Index of Need, a postnatal depression assessment and the history of the family.

Table 5.2 Record of parents' attributions about their infant observed during home visits

1. Attributions: (how the parents speak about and to the infant).		
Frequently positive	Occasionally positive	Rarely positive
Mother Father		

b) Perceptions

The parents' perception about their baby is another area of observation that can provide the community nurse with an understanding of how the parents feel. This involves reality-testing and is based on the parents ability to understand their infant's developmental pattern. Some parents expect a two-month-old to sleep throughout the night or a one-year-old to be fully toilet trained. Examples of areas in which parents can be very unrealistic about what the baby requires in terms of care and protection include:

- awareness of the child's nutritional needs as they grow
- the change in texture in the diet during the first year
- the baby's need for stimulation and play
- their need to be monitored throughout the day
- safety in the home once the baby starts to be mobile
- control of pets in the home with a baby around.

One mother thought that her baby would wake up and demand feeds, so would let her sleep throughout the night at two months of age without any night feeds. As the baby was particularly quiet and undemanding, she was getting less and less feeds and losing weight, as her mother would not feed her unless she cried. Despite this being pointed out by her health visitor the baby's weight did not improve as the mother was pleased not to be disturbed and wanted to get on with her own interests in the day. Eventually they were admitted to a mother and baby unit where the mother could learn how to understand and meet her baby's needs and to feed her appropriately.

Assessing both parents' perceptions is important as the father can influence what the mother thinks and does with her baby. A parent may not want having a baby to change their lives in any way and continue to live as if nothing has happened.

Unrealistic and distorted expectations of the infant's abilities can influence a parent's attitude towards discipline and punishment. They may have unrealistic expectations about developmental stages and the baby's level of independence. As described in Chapter 4, maltreating parents often have more negative conceptions of their infant's behaviour than non-abusing parents and they perceive their infants to be more irritable and demanding (Browne & Saqi, 1987).

One mother was proud that she had been dry at the age of three months and therefore expected her three-month-old baby to pass urine if she held her over a pot after every feed. She became worried and angry when her baby wet her nappy and felt she was being naughty.

An eight-month-old baby was failing to gain weight and an observation of a meal at home demonstrated that the mother expected her child to self-feed entirely and gave her no help.

High expectations can lead a parent into punishing their infant whom they perceive as being lazy, disobedient or naughty. Soiling a nappy that has just been changed, being sick on clean clothes, making a mess while eating, getting food in their hair and dropping it on the floor can all cause parents to feel frustrated. However, some may inappropriately blame the infant for doing this deliberately to upset them. Abusive parents may see their infant's behaviour as a threat to their own self-esteem, which then elicits punishment and an insensitive approach to parenting (Browne & Saqi, 1987, 1988b).

A four-month-old boy was left in his cot to feed from his bottle, which was propped upon a cushion while his mother prepared a meal for the other children. When it fell down and he cried, she was cross with him for knocking the bottle over and shouted at him.

The aim of the discussion with the parents is to bring them back to a sense of reality and provide them with information to reduce their anxiety:

- How rigid are their views?
- Are they amenable to change?
- What is the risk to the child?

A 12-month-old boy who was just learning to stand up while holding onto furniture had discovered how to pull open the kitchen cupboards. He kept going to the one under the sink that had all of the cleaning fluids in and pulling them out on the floor. His mother tried to ignore it while she was talking, but when her attention was drawn to what he was doing she smacked him and said that she had repeatedly told him not to go in that cupboard and that he was being deliberately naughty. She had made no effort to move the bottles out of reach, nor was there any thought of putting child proof locks on the doors.

An assessment is made of the parents' perceptions, in terms of their realism, at each visit in the first year of life (see Table 5.3). This will help indicate whether the parents' change their perceptions of the infant as he or she grows older, or if they remain rigid. A continual pattern of negative perceptions needs to be viewed in the context of the Index of Need, a postnatal depression assessment and the history of the family.

c) Quality of Parenting

The qualities of an affectionate parent-child relationship were identified earlier in the chapter as sensitivity, cooperation, accessibility and acceptance. These four concepts are useful for assessing the overall relationship with the infant and overlap to some extent. However, each one has specific features that are important in understanding how parents are reacting to their baby. The way in which the parents talk about their baby and how they describe their feelings for the baby will demonstrate how in tune they are with their baby's needs. In practical terms, the health visitor can be reassured when the following descriptions of these four concepts are observed in a family.

- **Sensitivity** is the ability of the parents to accurately perceive and interpret the infant's attachment signals and respond to them promptly and

Table 5.3 Record of parents' perceptions about their infant observed during home visits

2. How parents perceive infant behaviour.			
	Mostly realistic	Occasionally realistic	Rarely realistic
Mother Father			

adequately. The parents need to be able to observe or notice the baby's signals and be attuned to them.

Sensitivity will most often be observed non-verbally. The parents will demonstrate this in their physical reaction to the baby's noises, movements and presence. A sensitive mother usually looks at her baby frequently, checks the baby and may smile at or kiss the baby while talking about them. Gentle touch, soothing movements, cuddling, anticipating the baby's needs or responding rapidly once the baby's communication is understood will all demonstrate sensitivity. The parent may imitate the baby's noises, or reflect the baby's facial expressions or movements. The parent will demonstrate an understanding of the baby's emotional state and respond appropriately. The parent's own emotional state will not interfere with their ability to respond.

The parents' sensitivity to the child's needs and their accurate interpretation of communication from the infant is evident in daily comments and interactions. This can include guessing what is wrong when the infant cries, and knowing that the baby may be hungry, tired or has wind, as well as realising that their baby needs play and stimulation. In addition, cuddling their baby and enjoying physical contact, soothing and calming their baby, and keeping the baby warm and appropriately dressed for the weather are also all indicators that the parent is aware of the baby's needs.

The response of the parent needs to be prompt and related to the developmental ability of the baby to wait, so that the baby does not start to build up high levels of frustration. The aim is not to overprotect the baby but to see that the parent is supporting the infant's growth towards autonomy and their growing ability to communicate. The baby's needs do have to fit in with family life and the demands of other family members.

- **Supportive/cooperative** behaviour is often demonstrated verbally when the parents explain the baby's behaviour and why it is behaving in a particular way. They do not blame the baby nor are they critical but demonstrate understanding and sympathy. Cries are interpreted for a reason and behaviour is seen in a positive light. The parents see themselves as helping the baby cope with the world; they are the mediators and provide a safe and secure environment for their infant.

Physically, the parents will enable the baby to interact with their environment at a developmentally appropriate level. They recognise when the infant needs help to attain a goal, like crawling or standing up. They help get the toy that the baby is reaching for, they will support them as they try to sit or crawl. They will show the baby new stimuli in order for the baby to learn. Being supportive and cooperative with their baby will be reflected in how they help the infant attain new milestones in development. They demonstrate how things work to the baby and talk to them about what is happening. They wait if the baby is overwrought and help the baby calm down before proceeding with dressing or bathing.

The young parents of a five-month-old boy seemed to take delight in taking toys out of their baby's reach. They would put him on the floor and as soon as he showed interest in moving towards a toy, they would move it further away in order to see him struggle to reach it and giggle. They said it would make him a fighter.

- **Accessibility** is demonstrated when parents show that they respond to their baby's communications. A parent who is preoccupied and unaware of their baby's needs either due to depression, mental health problems, or substance abuse, i.e. alcohol or drugs, is not accessible to their baby. A parent or primary care-giver being under the influence of mood altering drugs or medication leaves the baby at risk. Stressed and anxious parents may find the demands of the baby overwhelming and so they may cut off from his or her demands in order to protect themselves. The break down of a parental relationship, moving home, being made homeless or severe financial problems can all create situations where parents are so involved with their own problems that they are not available emotionally to their baby.

   Parents or carers also need to be in reasonably close proximity to the baby all of the day. They should be able to hear the baby cry and, if the baby is out of sight, they should check regularly to see that the baby is safe. Babies who are left unattended for long periods can become passive and undemanding as they give up on making demands that are continually not met. Remember the patterns of behaviour shown by the babies in Romanian orphanages where the level of accessibility to staff and carers was minimal.

One 18-year-old single mother, who had been thrown out of the parental home after having her baby, was homeless. She had thought that the baby would bring the baby's father closer but he had abandoned her after the birth and she was left all alone. She left the baby in the pram all day and did not show any desire to pick the baby up to cuddle it. She fed the baby by bottle while lying in the pram and even changed his nappy in there. She admitted that the baby had ruined her life and regretted ever having had it.

- **Accepting** behaviour by the parents demonstrates that they understand that the baby has its own needs. They recognise the limitations of the baby's communication skills and physical skills. Their standards and expectations of the baby's abilities and behaviour are reasonable. They understand that the baby is totally dependent on them for care and protection and cannot make decisions. The fact that babies cry and have a different sleep pattern to adults is understood and accepted. They recognise that their baby is not deliberately trying to annoy them by vomiting on clean clothes or soiling a clean nappy.

Parents who are accepting of their baby will demonstrate this by being aware of their baby's developmental needs. They respond appropriately to the baby's stage of development and recognise that the baby is continually changing. They are flexible in adjusting routines and appreciate each stage that the baby passes through. They accept the dependence but also allow the growth of independence when the infant is ready.

One mother of twin 12-month-old boys kept them immaculately clean and tidy. She would change them up to five times a day if one of them got dirty and always made sure that they had matched clothes. She would not let them go in the sand when in the park or out into the garden to play. She would not let them touch their food and kept the bowl away from them while spoon-feeding them. She was unable to appreciate their own need to experience their environment and explore. Their weight had fallen below the third percentile and she complained that they would not eat their food.

An assessment is made of the quality of parenting at each visit in the first year of life and this will provide a picture of whether the quality of parenting remains constant or changes over time (see Table 5.4). A continual pattern of poor quality parenting needs to be viewed in the context of the Index of Need, a postnatal depression assessment and the history of the family.

The health visitor can complete these records of observations during the course of each visit in the first year of life because all these parental behaviours are observable by the tenth–fifteenth day postnatally. Therefore, the CARE programme recommends that observations of parents' attributions and perceptions of infant behaviour, together with an assessment of the quality of parenting, should be undertaken during a minimum of four visits spread over the first year of life (i.e., 4–6 weeks, 3–5 months, 7–9 months and

Table 5.4 Record of quality of parenting observed during home visits

3. Quality of parenting: Primary care-giver to infant			
	Frequently	Occasionally	Rarely
1. Sensitive			
2. Supportive/cooperative			
2. Accessible			
3. Accepting			

12 months; see Appendices 3 and 4). A referral for high priority families with identified difficulties can be made at any time during the first year based on any one of the observations. The aim of the referral is to access additional support for families in need.

Work with the parents to correct misperceptions, improve attributions and increase the quality of parenting can take place via supportive counselling, linking parents into parent support groups and networks, or identifying specific therapeutic needs in conjunction with other primary mental health care services.

2. The Infant's Reactions to the Parents

An important and unique feature of the CARE programme is the emphasis placed on observing the development of the infant's attachment to the primary care-giver/parent (usually the mother). The importance of observing the infant to mother attachment formation has already been highlighted in Chapter 4.

A number of factors need to be taken into account when observing attachment formation behaviour between children and their care-givers, such as,

- Is the infant being observed in its familiar surroundings?
- Are you familiar with the infant or will the infant see you as a stranger?
- Is the care-giver relaxed or are there apparent stress factors that are overriding the situation, which will interfere with the parents' responses to the infant?

If the parent or infant is ill, or other unusual factors appear to be affecting the observation (e.g., the presence of an excitable or aggressive pet dog), it is important to return and make another visit in order to carry out an accurate and reliable observation at each of the four visits over the first year. This is essential when you have observed difficulties in the parent-child relationship so that your observations are not based on a one-off situation.

The health visitor needs to ensure that the baby is directly observed during a visit in interaction with the mother. Using the opportunity to weigh the baby is one way of asking permission to see the baby and wake it up. Asking to see the baby if it is not in the room allows the proud parent to show off their baby and most parents would be delighted to be asked.

The behaviours that are listed in Table 5.5 are easily observable by two months of age and can give some early indication about the type of care the infant has received. The lack of these characteristics can also indicate some physical problems, i.e., vision or neurological difficulties, so either way this baby will need to be followed up regularly and perhaps a referral may need to be made to a GP or paediatrician.

Table 5.5 Early indications of infant attachment behaviour to the primary care-giver (4–6 weeks)

a) **Infant behaviour to care-giver at 4–6 weeks (specify who is primary care-giver: i.e., mother, father or other)**		
Frequently	Occasionally	Rarely
1. Smiles at care-giver		
2. Quietens when picked up by care-giver		
3. Responds to care-giver's voice		
4. Eye contact and scans care-giver's face		
5. Settles in care-giver's arms		

If problems are being detected in the baby's emotional response to the carer, then the health visitor needs to explore with the mother how she is feeling about caring for the baby, what the problems are for her and what would help her. Misperceptions can be corrected quickly and easily if they are approached early and rapidly. Helping the mother to understand what the health visitor is looking for and why is one way of teaching the mother about the needs of her baby. This is not a secretive assessment process or a one-off observation aimed at catching out parents. It should be a collaborative process that enables parents to openly discuss their difficulties and feelings and work with the health visitor to solve them before they get worse.

The health visitor's observations of the attachment formation behaviour shown in the 3–5-month-old infant can provide some very positive feedback about the infant (see Table 5.6). Drawing the mother's attention to the fact that the baby is watching her movements can be very informative and positive to most parents, who may not have noticed it. However, this information can be interpreted in a negative way to a mother who is having problems with attachment herself. She may see this as 'keeping an eye on her' or 'being nosey' in a way that is restrictive and intrusive, or that 'he's only looking for more food' rather than appreciating her. If the health visitor picks up the baby then a positive comment about mother being able to soothe the baby much better while handing the baby back to the mother is again positive feedback to the mother. However, a mother who is troubled may perceive this negatively and feel that the baby is always being dumped on her to sort out. Checking with the mother what her feelings are in these situations is crucial to understanding what is happening in the relationship. For example, what does the mother feel like when the baby does soothe and settle in her arms? Helping the mother persevere in soothing the baby by cuddling rather than putting the baby down may help her experience a first positive emotion

Table 5.6 Indicators that infant attachment to the primary care-giver is developing (3–5 months)

b) Development of attachment behaviour 3–5 months (specify who is primary care-giver: i.e., mother, father or other)			
	Frequently	Occasionally	Rarely
1. Turns head to follow care-giver's movement			
2. Responds to care-giver's voice with pleasure – windmill movements of arms/kicking legs			
3. Imitates 'speaking' to care-giver by moving lips in response to care-giver			
4. Shows preference to being held by care-giver by settling and quieting			

of coping and being capable as a mother. Helping her feed a fractious baby who cannot latch on easily to the nipple or the bottle can create a dramatic improvement in emotional relations between the mother and baby. Giving her support, encouragement and praise will help her feel appreciated and that she can be a good mother.

Looking for the reciprocal physical movements and noises between mother and baby can be fun and exciting to see. Babies will often mirror their mother's movements with slight time delay but if a mother is rushed and thinking only of the jobs she has to do, she will often miss this interchange. Taking time to watch and play can help develop the attachment as the mother starts to understand what the baby is doing.

By 7–9 months, attachment behaviour is becoming clearer (see Table 5.7). Infants usually want close proximity to their mothers, particularly if the mother is moving around. Mothers report not being able to leave the room or even go to the toilet without their baby crying or following them. By 12 months, most infants are wary of strangers and generally do not go up to strangers and want to be picked up. They may tolerate a stranger holding them but tend to go quiet and do not explore to the same extent that they will on their parents' laps. If the baby approaches the health visitor and wants to be picked up, although the health visitor may feel personally very pleased, this may not be a good indicator for the infant's attachment to his mother or carer. If the mother goes to work then the baby will make an attachment to a primary care-giver and can develop multiple attachments

Table 5.7 Infant attachment formation in the making (7–9 months and at 1 year)

c) **Attachment in the making at 7–9 months and at one year (specify who is primary care-giver: i.e., mother, father or other)**			
	Frequently	Occasionally	Rarely
1. Shows preference for primary care-giver			
2. Demonstrates some distress when left by primary care-giver			
3. Confident to explore – crawls away from primary care-giver, turns			
4. Relaxed, 'comforted' when held by primary care-giver			

to other carers, but they will still be wary of strangers. They show definite preference for the face of a primary care-giver over others. Explaining to parents that it is a positive sign of good attachment can be helpful when they feel embarrassed that the infant always cries when grandparents visit infrequently.

THE FINAL OBSERVATION AND ASSESSMENT OF NEED

This is the time to recap on all of the observations throughout the year and to think about the progress that the parents have made in coping with their new baby. This is the time that a decision will be made as to whether the case needs to be kept active for the following year or can be placed in the Inactive Caseload group and no regular further visiting planned. Nevertheless, the parents should be invited to make contact via the telephone or clinic with an 'open door' policy.

At the 12-month visit, the following assessments need to be undertaken and recorded:

- The parents need an opportunity to revisit the Index of Need and change some of the details or reflect on changes that have occurred during the year which may influence their future needs.
- A final assessment of the parents' attributions, perceptions and quality of parenting is conducted.
- A final rating of the infant's quality of attachment formation is conducted (see Table 5.8). This is based on indicators that may suggest the formation of a secure or insecure attachment, *but it is NOT an assessment of the*

Table 5.8 Indicators that a secure attachment between the infant and the care-giver has formed at 12 months

Indicators of secure attachment formation at 12 months			
	Frequently	Occasionally	Rarely
1. Seeks social interaction and physical contact with parent			
2. Actively plays in presence of parent			
3. Relaxed and happy in presence of parent			
4. Easily reassured by parents in front of a stranger			
5. Uses parent as a secure base to explore from			
6. Initially wary of strangers			

security of the attachment between the infant and the care-giver. This can only be done using separation and reunion episodes by qualified practitioners in the home or a strange situation (see Ainsworth et al., 1978).

Many cases will have grey areas of concern where the situation and the relationship between the parents and infant are not ideal. It is important to discuss these cases with colleagues and supervisors in order to clarify your assessment and thinking about the case and to make a decision about how best to help the family.

Cases of real concern will need to be referred to social services and the appropriate referral forms completed. Discussion and planning of this with parents will be a culmination of the year's work and will have developed out of facilitating them in recognising the needs that they have. Some parents will accept the referral to social services as a good way of helping them access more services while others may fearfully or forcefully reject it. The health visitor must keep the needs and safety of the child in mind when going against parents wishes. The referral to social services is not necessarily planned with the aim of removing the child but is to engage other professionals and services in supporting the family with their parenting task.

The observation of the emotional development and attachment of parent and child also takes places in the health promotion context. The total welfare of the child needs to be taken into account and so a final assessment of other welfare factors also needs to be conducted. Therefore, both during and following the fourth home visit assessments, the health visitor should fill out the completion summary section of Form B (see pages 180–183, Appendix 4). These evaluations are adapted from Herbert (1991) and involve an assessment and overall rating of

- physical care: safety, feeding, shelter, cleanliness and appearance of the infant
- responsive care: how sensitive and appropriate the parents' responses are to the infant and whether the responses are consistent and attuned
- psychological care: affection, security, guidance and control, stimulation and promotion of independence.

THE TIME TO BE CONCERNED

All parents complain about their babies at some time. No-one is happy having their life disrupted, no sleep and having to cope with crying babies. However, most families can balance the negative with the positive side of having a baby and do love their infant despite the difficulties. Negative comments can be checked out against positive comments; the ratio of positive to negative comments should always be higher (i.e., more positive than negative comments). Intermittent life stresses may create more strain for a period but this may have gone by the next visit. The baby may go through a difficult crying phase but this is resolved by the next visit. Using the observational guide, the health visitor can think through what she has heard and seen at each visit and determine whether there is improvement, no change or deterioration and this can be discussed openly with the parents. This also needs to be viewed in the context of any early interventions that have been tried and offered. The effectiveness of these early interventions and the parents' satisfaction and compliance with the strategy for support are important indicators of a prognosis for change when improvements in parenting are required in the best interests of the child. For example, if it takes three or more attempts to visit the infant in the home environment after agreeing an appointment with the parents, this is an indicator that would immediately place the family in the high priority group for support and services.

However, it is important to seek guidance from your supervisor in the following circumstances because the infant may be at risk of harm and the family is in high priority for need of additional support and services:

- The Index of Need score is 5 or more.
- The parental attributions about their baby have been rarely positive, i.e., the parent
  - has persistently denigrated or blamed the baby
  - ascribed inherent badness to the child
  - belittled or mocked the baby
  - has shown lack of eye contact with the baby, shown severe facial expressions or sneered at the baby
  - handled the baby roughly
  - purposefully and regularly ignored the baby's distress or demands.

- The parent's perceptions of their infant were rarely or only occasionally realistic, i.e., they
  - failed to recognise the baby's individuality and psychological boundaries
  - continually put their own needs first above the emotional needs of the baby
  - failed to acknowledge or accommodate to the baby's personality, worth or needs
  - attempted to modify the baby's personality coercively.
- The quality of the parenting was rarely or only occasionally positive, i.e., the parents
  - used harsh discipline or over control
  - terrorised through threats of severe physical punishment
  - used threats of abandonment
  - isolated or confined the infant
  - put the infant in frightening situations
  - disciplined by retaliation
  - were unpredictable
  - have shown inconsistent expectations
  - presented contradictory messages to the infant.
- The indicators for infant attachment behaviours and secure attachment formation to the primary care-giver are poor.
- The overall rating at 12 months for the parents' physical care of the infant is poor.
- The overall rating at 12 months for the parents' responsive care of the infant is poor.
- The overall rating at 12 months for the parents' psychological care of the infant is poor.

In such circumstances, it is necessary to consider a partnership plan between the parents and the health visitor that may involve a referral to social services or other health services (e.g., GP, paediatrician). The continual support of the health visiting service and voluntary groups may also be required. Therefore, the last page of the CARE programme form B (page 183, Appendix 4) is a completion summary of suggested referrals, together with a decision about further case management beyond one year. This decision will indicate whether routine surveillance (primary prevention) is continued through an 'open door' policy. Alternatively, the family will be offered prolonged active case management with intervention possibly involving referral to other agencies (secondary prevention).

6

CASELOAD MANAGEMENT

The CARE approach to managing cases in the first year of life creates a structure for record keeping which is crucial for effective communication with other agencies involved with the family or within the primary health care services. This structure should not end at the end of the first year of life, but should provide a basis for thinking and planning about the needs of the child older than one year. The relatively 'intensive' nature of the health visiting programme within the first year cannot continue indefinitely, so the health visitor does need to make a decision about any continuing needs of the child and family in conjunction with the parents. The end of year assessment reflects the Index of Need scores as well as the observational data collected by the health visitor during the year. From this, the health visitor can categorise the caseload and decide which cases will require further resources.

PROBLEMS OF IDIOSYNCRATIC CASE LOAD STRUCTURE

Effective caseload management and record keeping is an essential part of the community nurse's role. Historically, the method of organising a caseload has rested on the health visitor responsible for managing the caseload. The choice of organisation has often derived from what was taught in training or from fieldwork experience and colleagues. This has led to idiosyncratic approaches to caseload management and note keeping with no uniformity across clinics, services, districts or areas.

Problems arising from this approach include:

- ineffective communication
- loss of information
- an inability to trace cases
- an inability to pass on information to other professionals who become involved

- prioritising of cases that are unfamiliar can be difficult
- quality standards and audit can be more difficult and time consuming to complete
- data collection for comparison between clinics and districts is more difficult.

Children and their families who move regularly or have no fixed address can move ahead of their notes by several months. This can cause considerable problems for the new services and creates a break in service delivery. Similarly, staff who change jobs or who go off sick can create a problem for remaining colleagues who need to pick up their cases and are unfamiliar with the filing system in a particular caseload. Children may be at risk if information is not easily accessible or communicable.

The purpose of a structured approach to caseload management is:

- To enable a uniform approach in collecting data across the whole district.
- To base the approach on evidence-based practise.
- To identify agreed categories of work that health visitors can use effectively and have recognisable health gain outcomes based on evidence-based practice.
- To ensure that continued care can be delivered to children and their families should long-term sickness or uncovered caseloads arise.
- To ensure that audit can occur.
- To enable clinical governance and assessment of outcome.

All caseloads should aim to have a method of readily identifying:

- its characteristics
- high priority work
- areas of 'need'.

The advent of Parent Held Records and computer databases has started to produce the beginnings of corporate district approaches to organising caseloads.

The CARE programme aims to identify a method of evaluating 'concern' for the welfare of a child against which professional judgements can be made in partnership with the parents. The factor causing the concern should be specifically identified and the rights of the child should always be the primary concern (Children Act, 1989, 2004). Nevertheless, the rights of the parents are important and working in partnership with parents is essential. Where the professional concern is in conflict with parental rights (e.g., the child is removed under an Emergency Protection Order), the parents may be reluctant to engage in the care planning process. However, they must be encouraged to do so and reassured that the ultimate aim is always to try to reunite families, where possible.

All interventions whether directly by the health visitor or indirectly by referral to other community services must be evaluated in relation to the outcome for the child. If the health visitor is not involved in an assessment of the intervention effectiveness, then it is her professional responsibility to obtain this information from those professionals carrying out the evaluation process.

In some cases, parents will be unable to respond appropriately to the intervention offered in a time frame that is suitable for the infant. A change in the parents' behaviour may be essential for 'good enough' childcare in order for the infant to develop optimally and return home. However, at the present time, the parents may be unable to make that change; for example, due to emotional needs and distress, current relationship difficulties and/or substance abuse and addiction. Some parental difficulties may require long-term intervention with unclear prognosis for change. Parents may also lack motivation or an understanding of the need to change, which may be a symptom of their parental difficulties. In such cases, child protection procedures are usually instigated and the health visitor should work as a part of a multi-disciplinary team to determine what is in the best interests of the child, both in the short and long term.

CHART OF SIGNIFICANT EVENTS

For all types of cases, each child's record should have a chart of 'significant events', which details important psycho-social factors that have occurred in relation to the child's welfare (see Table 6.1). This allows effective handover of care and can demonstrate the sequence of a pattern of events. It helps the

Table 6.1 Chart of significant events

Name					
Age					
Date of birth					
Address					
GP & address					
Date of significant event	Action	Referral to	Current concern	Outcome	Signed
1.					
2.					

health visitor inform and remind herself but also enables information to be shared rapidly and effectively with others. Significant events can include:

- Accident and emergency or hospital admissions.
- A pattern of non-attendance for appointments.
- Parental factors such as drug addictions, violence in the family, partnership breakdown, frequent housing moves.
- Referral to social services, Child Protection Case Conferences, the child's name being added or removed from the Register plus criteria.
- Concern raised by other professionals or the community, i.e., other parents, playgroup, nursery nurse, GP.
- Record of own concerns or referrals based on observation.
- Record handover of care to new colleagues.

STRUCTURE OF THE CASELOAD

For those community professionals managing their caseload following the care programme, it is recommended that their case records be divided into an

(a) Active caseload: 0–1 years
- All new births up to one year filed under month of birth.
- Records of siblings to be filed together with youngest child.
- Index of Need and observations of parent attributions, perceptions, quality of parenting and indicators of infant attachment development recorded over four visits to the home.
- Infants and their families who are of professional concern or who are identified as being in need or at risk of significant harm are transferred into the selective caseload (a marker should be placed in the original database/index system).

(b) Routine caseload: 1–5 years ('inactive' routine surveillance)
- All children at one year of age, where there are no professional concerns, transfer into this category.
- Cases filed alphabetically in relation to family name, although a method of identifying the 2.5 year assessments by date of birth should be maintained.
- An open door policy is maintained where parents are given relevant information for continuing to gain health advice via the child health clinics; information to the parents should include the telephone number of the health visitor/health clinic.
- Involvement is maintained until the age of five years or when they start school, when records will be transferred to the School Health Service.

- Children and their families who are of professional concern or who are identified as being in need or at risk of significant harm are transferred into the selective caseload (a marker should be placed in the original database/index system).

(c) Selective caseload: 0–5 years (prolonged active management)
- Any child aged 0–5 years who is of professional concern or who is identified as being in need or at risk of significant harm.
- Cases filed alphabetically in relation to family name, although a method of identifying the 2.5 year assessments by date of birth should be maintained.
- Depending on the care plan, home visits (rather than reliance on clinic visits or an open-door policy) are essential to monitor the child's safety, care and welfare, and to assess indirectly or directly the effectiveness of any intervention.
- Involvement is maintained as necessary, even when records are transferred to the School Health Service.

COMPOSITION OF THE SELECTIVE CASELOAD

All children should have care plans that clearly identify professional interventions, health gain outcomes and are subject to regular review. The time scale should be stated in the care plan. Time frames should be set for regular review of the care plan with team members and the reviews should be recorded, dated and signed in the professional record.

Where children fit the criteria for more than one category, they should be placed in the category where most concern or intervention exists. All of the children in the selective caseload are offered an enhanced health visiting service and/or other health and social service referrals.

Children with a Significant 'Index of Need'

In two communities in south-east England, the Index of Need score has been used with a threshold of 'six or more' (see Chapter 9 for threshold analysis). When this threshold is reached, it may generate concern amongst health professionals depending on whether there is visible presence of a good parent-infant relationship. Observations of parent attributions, perceptions, quality of parenting and indicators of infant attachment formation will help determine whether a good infant-parent relationship is acting as a buffer against a high Index of Need score (6 or more) reflecting significant family stress. Alternatively, even in the absence of a high Index of Need score, the professional judgement of the health visitor is that concern exists – this may be based on the behavioural observations alone.

In either event, the child and/or parent require a public health intervention outside of the core programme. Direct interventions by the health visiting service may involve sleep management, behaviour modification, toilet training, play stimulation, parenting skills training and/or help with postnatal depression. Indirect interventions involve referrals to other health and social service agencies for support related to, for example, mental health problems, substance addiction, a violent adult in the household, socio-economic and/or housing problems.

As above, each record should have a 'chart of significant events' at the front of the record that is kept updated. Every child should have a care plan with clearly defined interventions and health gain outcomes. There should be regular reviews of the care plan every 4–6 weeks that are dated in the care plan.

Interventions with mothers suffering from postnatal depression or mental illness will be aimed at supporting the mother through the crisis and ensuring the safety of the child. The health visitor will work in partnership with the Adult Community Mental Health team and will assist the Community Psychiatric Nurse (CPN) in their duty of care to the parents. The health visitor's prime concern is the capacity of the parent/carer to adequately protect and care for the infant, and meet their developing requirements. Clinical supervision must be built into the care plan when postnatal depression or mental illness in the family is a feature.

Children with a Diagnosed Disability or Health Need

These children will have Special Educational Needs and/or will be under periodic review by the paediatricians. They will have a key worker in social services. Again, each record should have a chart of significant events at the front of the record that is kept updated and every child will have a care plan. This should be reviewed at not less than six monthly intervals. The health visitor will contribute to the paediatric team assessment. Outcomes of the reviews should be recorded in the professional and child health record. The care plan should be forwarded to the School Nurse when the child enters the education system.

Children with Developmental Delay

These children require repeat developmental assessments or require nursery placement due to delay or are receiving other services to promote their development. As before, each record should have a chart of significant events at the front of the record that is kept updated. Each child will have a care plan that should be reviewed every eight–ten weeks and the outcomes recorded in the professional record and child health record. The aim is to enable the children to reach their full potential. Additional resources may need to be mobilised. If the child remains delayed despite interventions and will require Special Educational Needs at school age, then a transfer into the 'Disabilities' category will be appropriate.

Children Classified as 'In Need' Referred to Social Services

Children 'in need' will have a key worker in social services, but are not managed under child protection or children with disabilities teams. Again, each community nurse record should have a chart of significant events at the front of the record that is kept updated. Each child will have a formulated care plan, which includes the planned interventions of all of the professionals working with the family and will form the basis of shared information for social services review meetings. All planned interventions by the Health Visiting Service should have clearly identified health gain outcomes. The care plan should be reviewed at a minimum of four weeks and the outcome of the review should be recorded in the professional record. Clinical supervision must be specified in the care plan.

Children on the Child Protection Register

All children on the register will be subject to specific case management that is structured and managed through social services and entails staff from all agencies complying with the procedure outlined in 'Working Together to Safeguard Children' (Department of Health et al., 1999).

As described above, each record should have a chart of significant events at the front of the record that is kept updated and every child must have a care plan that reflects the identified piece of work the health visitor has contracted to undertake as a core group member. The care plan should be reviewed at a minimum of four weeks. It will form the basis of the shared information from core group meetings and child protection conferences, and should include the planned interventions of all professionals working with the child or family. A synopsis of the care plan review must be written in the child health record, the actual care plan can form part of the professional record. Child protection clinical supervision must be built into the care plan.

In a review of 200 consecutive child protection case conferences (Simpson et al., 1994), there was no primary care team input (attendance or written report) in 32% of cases by either the GP or the health visitor. As only one in ten child protection case conferences are attended by the GP, the health visitor should make sure that she is always in attendance to represent the primary health care team.

Children being 'Looked After' by the Local Authority

These children are in short-term or long-term foster care, awaiting adoption or have statutory orders, e.g., Emergency Protection Order or Care or Supervision Orders. Again, each record should have a chart of significant events at the front of the record that is kept updated, but this should also include the legal status of the child and who has parental responsibility (confirmed with the key worker). Children in long-term foster care or awaiting adoption may not require a care plan. However, children who remain Looked After with a plan to return to the main care-giver's home who originally caused concern for the child's welfare will need a care plan. If there is a care plan, there should be regular review at four–six weekly intervals and the outcomes of the review documented in the professional record. The progression of the care plan should be recorded in the child health record.

CHILDREN WHO TRANSFER OUT OF THE CASELOAD

Health visitors are generally notified of the removal of children from their caseload by:

- Child Health Records Department
- GP practice 'transfer in-out list'
- parents informing the health visitor
- other methods of informal information gathering.

Once the health visitor is aware of the movement of the family from their caseload, they should endeavour to transfer the record to the Child Health Department within one week. They should also liaise with colleagues in the receiving authorities in order to pass information to them that is relevant to the child's/family's continuity of service. The aim is for the child and family to receive a seamless service.

In a case of Child Protection, the health visitor should follow the guidance for Transfer of Records and inform the named nurse for Child Protection. It may also be appropriate to inform other professionals of the transfer of the case, particularly if the child or family was receiving a health visiting service from within the Selective caseload and a contractual piece of work that involved the expertise of other professional colleagues and key workers was being provided.

7

HOW TO HELP PARENTS IN THE BEST INTERESTS OF THE CHILD

WORKING TOGETHER WITH PARENTS

The 'partnership with parents' approach discussed in Chapter 2 is the basis for much of the community nurses' work that is carried out with families with young children. This collaborative approach creates a supportive and friendly atmosphere for parents to work out what they need and how to think about their problems. It is based on sharing the responsibility for participation and decision-making.

Deciding whether there are any problems is the first step. Some parents may not even realise that there is a problem or they may try to hide it because they are unsure of the security of their relationship with the community nurse, as well as what services can be offered to them in the way of help. Parents have to trust professionals so that they can fully express their feelings and not feel let down or judged adversely. However, they may have had a history of poor relationships with professionals, resulting in an 'us and them' situation. They may also have fears about the power of the health care professional or unfounded worries about the possibility of their child being removed from them, especially if they reveal inadequacies.

Therefore, health visitors need to assess whether parents understand and listen to what health professionals advise. Do they see health professionals working with them for the sake of their child or against them? Professionals working in the community should ask parents about the following during their introductory visit to facilitate a trusting relationship:

- What are parents' perceptions of a community nurse health visitor?
- What do they expect from their health visitor?
- Why do they think the health visitor comes to the family home?

In addition, the health visitor should impart the following information:

- An explanation of the health visiting role to support infants, children and families.
- The importance of visiting the home environment.
- How their health visiting service can help them (e.g., promotion of appropriate infant feeding, establishing infant care routines, prevention of accidents in the home).

The community nurse's authority and professional position can make some parents feel uncomfortable. The creation of a caring relationship with the parents will help combat many of these concerns and allow the parents to be more realistic about their worries.

The family should not feel stigmatised in any way and the community nurse should avoid the use of negative labels (such as 'high risk family') at all costs (Barlow et al., 2003). Rather, positive labels (such as 'family in priority') should be used. Most importantly, a high Index of Need score placing a family in priority for services does not mean that maltreatment of the child is inevitable. Discussing with the parents the factors that give them a high score on the Index of Need and suggesting ways in which intervention may help gives a high chance that adverse outcomes for the child and family will be prevented.

The Index of Need has been found by many community nurses to be an important way of demonstrating to parents the range of issues in which they are interested. It raises issues in the minds of the parents that may be important but that they had not considered would be important. The discussion about how they feel about their new baby may be the first time that someone has listened to them, rather than told them how lovely or difficult their baby is.

Joining with the parent and using 'we' instead of 'I' can be a sign that this is a joint process. Ways to express this can include the following:

- 'Let's think how we can work out what will be helpful for you in this situation'.
- 'We need to think about the best way of arranging care for your baby while you are at work, have you had any ideas?'
- 'We could consider linking you into a breast feeding group, how would you feel about that?'
- 'How can we make your home safe for an infant and toddler to freely explore without accidents?'

The role of the community nurse is to empower the parents and enable them to reach the services that they require. The health visitor is well informed about available services and how they are accessed, and is therefore able to help parents plan their own support. However, the community nurse's role is to make herself expendable in the long-term rather than foster dependence; parents can often choose what is best for them once they know what is available.

The community nurse also has knowledge about child health and development, which can help parents think about how to cope with normal behavioural and emotional issues in their family and with their baby. Health visitors know about the needs for 'good enough' parenting, as well as the needs of a child for a safe and protected environment. In addition, they know how attachments between parents and children develop and mature. Overall, therefore, community nurses are a fund of knowledge that the parents need to learn how to tap into and how to put it into practice. Professionals are not books where parents can look up a topic, but they can guide, prompt and challenge in an active manner that encourages the parents to try out a new approach. Community nurses can use this knowledge in an effective and supportive manner by:

- Helping parents manage their infant in a slightly different way.
- Pointing out how the baby's behaviour reflects theirs so that they understand the baby's communications better and see the baby as an active learner and anticipator.
- Helping them reflect on what the baby's cries might mean by watching and trying different reactions.
- Loosening up rigid expectations.
- Moving parents along the road to accepting responsibility for safety and hygiene.
- Helping parents generate solutions to problems themselves.

We all learn more effectively when we are ready for the information that we are being given. If the access to the knowledge is at times when we are most attuned to using it then we can learn very rapidly. However, anxiety, stress, distraction and disinterest all adversely affect the rate at which we learn. Therefore, although some parents will take the pieces of information that they want and use them very effectively, others will be unable to do so as they are distracted and preoccupied with other concerns.

MANAGING PARENTS' CONCERNS

New parents have a myriad of concerns about themselves and their baby. They worry about whether:

- they will be or are a good parent
- their own childhood problems will come back to haunt them
- their relationship with their own parents will affect how they relate to their baby
- their partner will stand the strain of caring for a baby.

They may have concerns about:

- their own health
- their baby's health
- their baby's development
- sleep problems
- feeding problems
- crying
- weight gain
- responsibility for child care and safety
- child care skills
- loss of personal freedom
- maintaining an intimate relationship with their partner
- financial resources
- work
- housing.

Often they will express some of these concerns openly, but others they will keep to themselves unless helped to express them. Facilitating parents to say how they feel is a necessary part of developing the working relationship. They cannot be helped unless they have expressed their concerns. Parents can feel guilty about a whole range of issues some of which may be irrelevant to the process of being a good parent, but guilt can undermine and disrupt how they respond effectively to their baby.

Some of the parents' concerns can be answered simply and easily, and the worry will disappear. However, other concerns may be deep seated and it may be necessary to enquire why the parent is worried about that now. The question asked by the parent may be tangential to the underlying concern and the alert community nurse needs to be aware that this is a leading question that could expose greater concerns underneath.

Other parents will readily express their concerns but do not want to listen to answers – they need to unload their anxiety or their stress and have a shoulder to cry on. Just being there for parents like this so that they can let out their feelings can be helpful and supportive and allow them to feel heard. Reflecting back to them what they say is an effective tool for allowing them to know they have been understood. Furthermore, the process of talking it out can help some parents clarify their thoughts and make a decision on their own.

Some parents want specific information, for example on how to manage feeding or sleeping problems. The way in which this is offered is critical in how effective it is. Whilst it is easy to tell parents what they should do, it is much more difficult to ensure that they carry out the advice effectively. We all have difficulty receiving advice at times and tend to modify it in the way that we want to. Therefore, it is important to be wary of giving specific instructions without understanding how the parents interpret it. It is usually far more effective to enable parents to come to the decision to change themselves (through discussion) and help them think through the problem and highlight the alternatives of action. Facilitating parents' own problem solving and decision-making skills empowers them to take control rather than just doing as they are told.

BUILDING ON STRENGTHS

Parents have considerable strengths that they bring to the task of caring for their children. Even with poor environmental circumstances, inadequate finances, unemployment and poor housing conditions, they can provide a caring and loving home. Others have good intentions but need support and training in how best to apply their strengths. They may recognise the areas they need help and support with and can be open to advice.

The skill of bringing out the positive aspects of parents' personalities, skills and behaviour involves recognising their strengths and pointing them out. This can be an enhancing experience for parents who have never received that type of attention previously. It builds up their self-esteem and self-confidence and as they feel better about themselves, they cope better with being parents. Praise is always far more constructive than criticism, it enables learning to take place rapidly and cooperatively. The 'teacher' is also seen in a positive light and it enhances the relationship between the professional and the parent. The community nurse needs to learn to look for good instances of parent-infant interaction, positive assessment of the current conditions, positive/caring statements about the baby and an optimistic or coping outlook to the future. Reinforcing these instances will increase the likelihood of their occurrence and improve the parents' outlook and behaviour. A nurturing relationship between the community nurse and the parents will facilitate the parents' ability to face problems and acknowledge where they need help, rather than avoid problems and hide the reality of the difficulties they are facing.

POSITIVE PARENTING AND
PARENT-CHILD ATTUNEMENT

The most recent approach to intervention with parent-toddler relationships that are high risk for maltreatment is parent-child attunement therapy (Dombrowski et al., 2005). This involves the use of an ear-piece ('bug') to feed-back to the parent whilst they are interacting with their toddler, watched by a therapist through a one-way mirror. The results have been promising as they demonstrated an increase in the number of positive interactions and have been shown to improve the quality of the parent-toddler relationship. However, this technique did not always result in positive change, which highlights the fact that treatment occurs within the context of a wider environment that will include stress factors for the family (Dumbrowski et al., 2005).

A more comprehensive approach is to offer different intensity of interventions matched to the needs of the child and family. This has been the principle of the Triple P – Positive Parenting Programme, for children aged 0–12 years and for teenagers. Triple P intervenes with individual, group or self-directed therapy at all levels of prevention: universal, targeted and specialist (Sanders & Cann, 2002; Sanders, Cann & Markie-Dadds, 2003). Therefore, Triple P is offered at five levels:

- Level 1: Universal Triple P – Media and promotional campaigns providing parenting information (e.g., 'Driving Mum and Dad Mad', ITV, 2005). This is primary prevention aimed at the whole population.
- Level 2: Selective Triple P – one to two sessions of brief consultation offered by health professionals in clinics and/or the home. The purpose is to give brief parenting advice through the use of 'tip sheets' on parenting issues, such as toileting, tantrums, feeding and sleeping. This is also primary prevention aimed at the whole population.
- Level 3: Primary Care Triple P – four sessions of parenting intervention with a community nurse in the clinic and/or home environment. This is aimed at parents who feel they need some help to cope with their child's behaviour and development. Workbooks, video and diaries are used to support these families, who may be low or high risk for child maltreatment. Hence this is both primary and secondary prevention.
- Level 4: Standard Triple P – this is intensive parent training (eight–ten sessions) offered by psychotherapists for families who are not coping with their child's behaviour and are at increased risk for harsh discipline and physical abuse or neglect. This is secondary prevention.
- Level 5: Enhanced Triple P – (ten–sixteen sessions) offered by psycho-therapists for an intensive family intervention programme when there are issues of maternal depression and/or difficulties in the parents' relationship, including violence. This is secondary prevention.

At tertiary level, families who have been identified as requiring treatment for potential child maltreatment, follow the 'Pathways Triple P' programme, which again offers levels 2–5 systematically. At each level, the underlying objective is to promote positive parenting using the following core principles (Sanders et al., 2003):

- *Ensuring a safe and engaging environment*: to prevent accidents and injuries in the home and allow the child to explore, experiment and play safely.
- *Creating a positive learning environment*: the parent is taught to assist their child to learn and problem-solve for themselves in a positive and constructive way. In addition, the aim is to enhance parental sensitivity to the child's attempts to communicate, the parent being 'the child's most important teacher' (Sanders et al., 2003; p. 162).
- *Using assertive discipline*: offering parents safe and appropriate alternatives to coercive and ineffective disciplining, e.g., shouting, threatening, physical punishment. The parents are given a range of alternative procedures for responding to non-compliant behaviour to use in the home and community settings (e.g., ground rules; planned ignoring; discussing rules with children; directed discussion for rule-breaking; giving clear, calm and age-appropriate requests; logical consequences; quiet time and time out).
- *Having realistic expectations*: through discussion, parents are encouraged to develop realistic goals, developmentally appropriate expectations and reappraise negative perceptions of their child.
- *Taking care of oneself as a parent*: it is recognised that parents need to take care of themselves so that they are in a position to fulfill their role as care-givers. Parents are encouraged to develop coping strategies for managing stress and feelings, such as anger, anxiety, low self-esteem and depression.

The advantage of the Triple P programme and its varied delivery modalities is that it has a wide potential reach to many families with different problems, including children with disabilities (Stepping Stones Triple P), using a multi-disciplinary approach. The programme has been adapted to several cultures and languages, currently running in twelve countries. It has a strong evaluation base with over 20 years of research. A review of the effectiveness of Triple P as a multi-level intervention strategy can be found in Sanders (1999).

However, no intervention programme lasts forever. Parents need to become self-sufficient and independent of their therapists so that they learn to solve problems themselves. Therefore, Triple P uses a self-regulation framework to promote parental self-sufficiency, self-efficacy and self-management by the end of the intervention. Parents who benefit from the intervention begin to trust their own judgement and use their new skills to solve problems related to the management of the child. As a consequence of therapy, parents should be able to self-monitor their parenting and set their own standards and goals. Eventually the parent attributes improvements in the parent-child relationship and the child's behaviour to their own actions and decisions, rather than changes in the child or the environment. This often enhances parental self-esteem and consequently parental sensitivity, which is important for fostering secure attachments.

FOSTERING SECURE ATTACHMENTS

Good attachments occur when a parent can feel and show love towards their baby. When parents recognise that the baby is an independent individual with needs that have to be met, they can empathise with their baby. The infant develops a secure attachment when the parent is consistent and caring, provides stimulation and interaction, and is warm and sensitive to its needs and communication.

The parents need to realise the importance of creating time to enjoy playing and having fun with their baby. A baby is not just hard work and chores but gives pleasure by making parents smile, feel proud, laugh and be fascinated. Carrying, cuddling, soothing and rocking all involve the parents in close physical interaction that helps them understand their baby better. Watching their baby's expressions, listening to its different sounds, observing its movements and behaviour will enable parents to learn how to interpret more accurately their baby's communications. This takes time and patience. Parents have to learn to make space and time in their lives for their baby. They cannot carry on living the life they lived prior to the birth. Accommodation to the baby's needs and presence are an important adjustment that parents need to make.

Sensitive care giving is defined by the mother's prompt response that is also consistent and appropriate to her baby's signals. In turn, watching her baby and learning how her baby behaves can open a parent's eyes. It is often possible to observe interactional synchrony in securely attached parents and infants. This is an 'emotional dance' with mutually rewarding interactions and matching emotional states. Mothers will reflect the movements, sounds and facial expressions of the baby and the baby will do this back to the mother. They take turns and both gain satisfaction from the communication. A mother who is over-stimulating her baby may be intrusive and unresponsive to the baby's signals, leading to inconsistent care and a frustrating experience for both of them with little feedback. Similarly, a mother who is rigid or over-controlling will have trouble moderating her own wishes and needs to those of the baby. Helping these mothers relax, have fun and enjoy their baby without an ulterior motive or plan can be a hard task. They need guidance in slowing down, watching, and being led by their baby in the interaction.

A mother with postnatal depression may have difficulty in recognising the effect of her behaviour on her baby. However, postnatal depression can lead to emotional 'flatness' and a preoccupation with one's own feelings, both of which can interfere with the mother's attachment to her baby. Gaining some personal help with her depression from the GP or local mental health service in conjunction with support from the community nurse (whose primary concern is the care and welfare of the baby), is an ideal combination. Home visiting allows the community nurse to observe directly the quality of the relationship between mother and baby and intervene directly when appropriate. Providing the mother with emotional support in her role as a parent is an important preventative role. The community nurse can mobilise local community resources or involve other family members to help for short periods; the aim being to support the parent-infant relationship, not to be judgemental or critical. Working with the mother to think about her needs and those of her baby during the period of postnatal depression and helping her and her partner make decisions about what help is required is a facilitative process.

Fostering good attachments is a basic building block for the child's later mental health and other attachments later in life. The pattern of attachment that is established in the first year of life will remain fairly stable until the teenage years unless something significant interferes. Attachment patterns tend to repeat themselves through the generations. A mother who is insecurely attached has an increased likelihood of raising a child who is also insecurely attached and often intervention is needed to break the pattern. Even a brief intervention can break the pattern so the importance of preventative work in the first year should not be understated. However, it is also important to recognise that attachment patterns can change over the lifespan, with adult attachment style being more dependent on their relationship with their partner than their early attachment figure (Cowan & Cowan, 2001).

Some parents need help to reflect on their own early experiences of being parented. It may be the first time in many years that they have looked back on their childhood and tried to understand what happened to them. It may be painful and they may feel angry or distressed, but it can help them think about their relationship with their own baby and how they want it to be different. The way parents view their own childhood is a more important predictor of attachment than the reality of the childhood experiences. Translating good intent into action is a different matter and some parents will need a lot of support to deal with the emotions evoked by being a parent and by problems in their own adult relationships. Helping them think about what it is to be a good parent takes them beyond thoughts about buying new toys or clothes for the baby and into thinking about what the baby needs in terms of emotional support, stimulation and care.

Some parents benefit from direct training in breast feeding support or with baby massage classes. Helping the parent understand the baby's signals and getting to know their baby is a vital part of learning about how to manage. Giving themselves time and space to enjoy playing with or massaging their baby, allows parents to acknowledge that the baby has special needs for personal attention during the day and cannot just be treated as yet another chore on top of the housework or daily jobs. Linking these parents into local baby massage classes, parent support groups or breast-feeding support groups can all help create an environment when the needs of the baby and the mother are addressed directly.

A common irritant to parents is persistent crying, usually associated with colic or teething during infancy. It is well established that, when the infant is in distress, the most effective response to calm the infant is to hold it in your arms and comfort it (Dunn, 1977). Contrary to common myths (e.g., 'the Contented Little Baby' book), responding immediately to a crying infant should result in the baby crying less in the longer term, rather than more (Bell & Ainsworth, 1972). Cross-cultural studies on parents who carry their children close to their bodies have shown that this is associated with the extent of crying in infants: those carried most, cry least (Ainsworth, 1977).

Parents can learn about their baby by carrying them close to their bodies in a baby sling so that they come to know their baby's movements, wake and sleep cycles, noises and communications. The immediacy and intimacy of the contact helps some mothers rapidly to respond in a more predictable manner. Of course just using a baby sling/carrier and not responding to the baby's needs does not help particularly. The most important feature is the response of the mother to the baby, not just the carrying. Indeed, one study provided mothers with baby carriers during the first months of life and found that the process of being carried closely had a significant effect on the infant's attachment security, above and beyond that attributable to an increase in maternal sensitivity (Anisfeld et al., 1990).

A review of sixteen studies found that interventions that were effective in changing parental sensitivity to the infant's attachment cues were effective in enhancing the quality of the parent-infant attachment relationship (Ijzendoorn et al., 1995). The studies fell into two types:

- Behaviourally orientated support aimed at increasing the mother's sensitivity to her baby's behaviour.
- Reflective interventions aimed at improving the mother's attachment by reflecting on her own childhood attachment to her parents (Lieberman et al., 1991).

They found that brief, focused preventative interventions that targeted parent sensitivity and behaviour were more effective than long-term broad-based interventions. For example, a short intervention with mothers involving three or four home visits, when the infants were aged between seven and nine months, enhanced maternal sensitivity and infants' secure attachments. This was achieved by helping the mothers adjust to their babies' unique cues, particularly negative signals like crying, and to stimulate playful interaction (Van den Boom, 1991).

Similarly, studies aimed at disadvantaged pregnant women with low social support have found that one year of home visits by community nurses resulted in the mothers' being rated as more sensitive and competent (Barnard et al., 1988), and infants were identified as being more securely attached to their mothers (Jacobsen & Frye, 1991; Lyons-Ruth et al., 1990). These changes were achieved by the health visitor supporting the women in their daily lives. They provided a role model and talked about the pregnancy, preparation for the baby, the mother's expectations, developmental milestones and health concerns, as well as the kinds of activities that mothers and infants enjoy doing together.

A more specific preventative project for low income parents who had sick premature babies, commenced when the babies were in hospital and progressed onto regular home visits. The home visitor tried to develop a trusting and supportive relationship, provided concrete assistance and encouraged the development of observational skills towards the baby. They found that there was increased maternal involvement and an increased level of reciprocal interaction at nine months of age (Beckwith, 1988).

Attachment theory (Bowlby, 1969) would predict long-term benefits from fostering secure attachments between the infant and mother following birth. Indeed, the long-term effects of home visits to families with newborns have been highlighted through evaluating a two-year community nurse home visitation programme in Denver, Colarado (Kitzman et al., 1997, 2000; Olds et al., 1997, 1998). The research was conducted over a 15-year period and, on follow-up, a number of significant differences were found between those families randomly selected for visitation and those families with a newborn who were not. In summary, the visited families showed the following differences:

- lower rates of child abuse and neglect
- fewer births after the first child for unmarried women
- less family aid received
- fewer problems with alcohol and drugs
- fewer arrests by police.

These differences were found for both parents and children up to 13 years after the visitation had ceased and, hence, are probably related to the development of secure attachments as a result of early intervention by the community nurses. Nevertheless, many parent and child difficulties require additional and specialist health and social services care at a secondary and tertiary level of prevention (e.g., Child and Adolescent Mental Health Services Tiers 2 and 3). Thus, through the work of his or her primary health care team, the community nurse must engage in a multi-disciplinary network of professionals.

However, recent research that randomly assigned families who had already physically abused or neglected a child to either a) a standard health care intervention or b) standard health care plus home visitation by community nurses over a two year period, found that there was little effect on the reoccurrence of maltreatment to the child (MacMillan et al., 2005). This indicates that home visits by community nurses cannot be used as a treatment for maltreating families, which require a multi-disciplinary team approach. Rather the value of health visiting is to prevent maltreatment beginning by adequate support and referral for factors associated with increased risk.

WORKING TOGETHER WITH PROFESSIONALS

Interagency collaboration and cooperation for the welfare of children and families have been facilitated by the existence of Area Child Protection Committees (ACPCs) and Multi Agency Public Protection Panels (MAPPPs). However, child care and protection practices have been found to be variable across the nation. Sufficient levels of appropriately qualified staff and a lack of consistent local service planning have contributed to this variability. Thus, the Joint Chief Inspector's Report on Arrangements to Safeguard Children observed that 'many staff from all agencies were confused about their responsibilities and duties to share information about child welfare concerns with other agencies and were not confident about whether other agencies shared information with them' (Dept of Health, 2005, p. 4).

Under the Children Act (2004), it is the duty of Local Authorities to promote cooperation between professionals from different agencies, in order to make arrangements to care for and protect children in partnership with parents. In this respect, Local Authorities will set up 'Local Safeguarding Children Boards' involving key professionals from partner agencies. It is expected that Primary Care Teams (PCT) will take part in this initiative to safeguard and promote the welfare of children. It is proposed that index databases containing basic information about children will improve information sharing between agencies. It is suggested that the CARE programme may go some way in fulfilling this requirement for primary care teams. The 'Every Child Matters' initiative (DfES & DoH, 2004) intimates that PCTs have a duty to cooperate with other agencies to provide community health services that achieve the following:

- Promote children's welfare with effective procedures in place.
- Prevent the impairment of children's health and development.
- Prevent children from being abused or neglected.
- Act to protect children from being harmed or from suffering further harm and collaborate to provide services for the child and family.
- Identify children who may be at risk of significant harm and follow the local procedures for referral to social services or the police.
- Ensure that where concerns exist, they participate in a timely and thorough multi-agency assessment (led by social services).
- Contribute to a comprehensive child and family assessment, as appropriate.
- Contribute to case conferences and reviews.
- Ensure staff use effective systems to record their work with children and carry out caseload analysis.
- Ensure that clinical governance arrangements cover all aspects of child health and safety.

The government guidelines also encourage common assessments where possible and the CARE programme would suggest that this is feasible for community nurses (i.e., midwives, health visitors, school nurses and community psychiatric nurses).

The skills of midwives and health visitors are best applied to preventative approaches, such as the promotion of positive parenting in families. However, it is important to recognise that home visits by community nurses do not occur in isolation. The provision of primary care and community health services may coincide with the education of parents through their children attending pre-school and school, information received via media campaigns and contacts with telephone help lines. Indeed, the Triple P programme has used local networks to reinforce positive parenting programmes offered by the health sector. In parallel, programmes have been developed for use in the media, schools and the workplace (see Figure 7.1). Within this ecological model of intervention, parents and teachers both attend programmes to learn about the same positive parenting skills. Hence, the children's experiences at home and at school are the same.

Using Local Networks and Resources

The primary care team and community nurse health visiting service may provide a number of in-house services, depending on personnel and

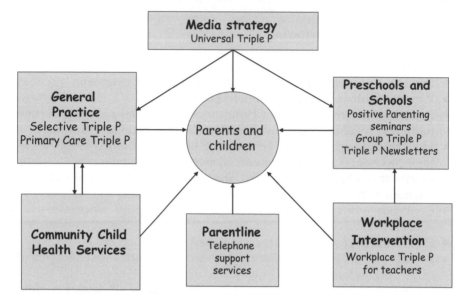

Figure 7.1 Ecological model of intervention
From Sanders, Cann & Markie-Dadds, 2003.

financial resources available. Indeed, some health visitors may wish to spe-
cialise in providing a service in their area of interest. However, some of these
primary and secondary prevention services may be offered in conjunction
with other professionals within the health sector through a cross-referral
system, including:

- breast feeding support group
- postnatal care and parental support group
- baby massage group
- clinics for advice on children's sleep and bedtime
- positive parenting skills
- postnatal depression group
- parent survivors of abuse group.

The voluntary sector also runs support groups for new parents, some of
which are provided by charities, religious organisations or ethnic minority
groups. The community nurse may act as a facilitator enabling and encouraging reluctant or socially anxious mothers to attend a group. This can
include helping mothers with transport, attending a group with a new
mother, arranging translators and identifying a support worker or another
parent in the community.

Local authority links and referrals to social services may be required to arrange a playgroup, alternative day care for the infant, a nursery placement or appropriate housing. This is particularly important for single and/or homeless mothers. The community nurse may also provide important evidence to the Housing Department, Electricity or Water Boards on behalf of poor families. For example, housing conditions and unhealthy environments that affect the family should be of concern to the community nurse, social worker and Housing Department. Advice on how to access the Citizen's Advice Bureau for help with debt counselling, legal advice and housing rights is necessary for some parents. Other local support groups include Bereavement counselling, Disability, Parent's Action, Single Parent Association, Gingerbread, Give a Lift Scheme, Children's Society and Home Start volunteers to befriend new mothers.

Each social services department has a list of voluntary agencies and often coordinate the Local Association of Voluntary Service in each area. Pooling knowledge of these resources among the community nurses provides useful knowledge to everyone and is of benefit to all families.

In addition, the private sector should not be forgotten. Child carers, playgroups and nurseries are mostly in the private sector. Some parents who are able to pay for services or have private health insurance will opt into the private sector and so it is important for community nurses to know of the available private services in their area. This should include psychotherapists and counsellors for alcohol addiction, substance abuse, adult survivors of sexual abuse, debt counselling and legal advice. Private health insurance may also give quick access to child psychologists, psychiatrists and paediatricians. GPs often know of the private sector provision and so advice from them can be valuable.

REFERRING ON FOR SPECIALIST HELP

A number of children will need an NHS referral to specialist or secondary statutory services in the area. This will include social services, specialist paediatric services and Child Adolescent Mental Health Services (CAMHS). For the parents, the adult mental health, addiction or substance abuse services may be required, together with social and probation services that may offer domestic violence intervention programmes. The routes of referral, the referral system process and the types of problems suitable for referral need clarification and agreement at regional level prior to implementing any screening or assessment procedure. The CARE programme enables clarity within the referral system and enables the community nurse to be clear and concise about the concerns for the child and their family. This is particularly important for child protection cases.

The responsibility for the well-being and protection of children must be shared across all agencies and professional groups (Dept of Health, 1991, 1999) and effective communication between agencies and professionals is essential to keep children safe (Dept of Health et al., 2003). This is because it is now well established that the care and protection of children is influenced by social exclusion, domestic violence, parent mental illness and substance addiction.

8

CHILD PROTECTION

Child protection is generally regarded as a broad concept concerned with the prevention of significant harm to children. Hence, it is concerned with the prevention of failure to thrive, accidents in the home and the maltreatment of children.

It has been estimated that 3–5% of infants under one year of age who are hospitalised are diagnosed as having failure to thrive (FTT; Iwaniec, 2004). It is often difficult to determine whether the cause of the growth failure is biological/organic or for psychosocial reasons. The prevalence of organic FTT ranges between 17% and 58%, and for non-organic FTT the range is from 32% to 58% of samples (Spinner & Siegel, 1987). Therefore, community nurses' monitoring of height, weight and head circumference during the first year of life is essential for the protection of children. If the infant's weight falls below the third percentile for three months or more, this should cause significant concern.

Community nurses have an obvious role to advise parents on how to prevent accidents and make the home environment safe, as the infant develops mobility. Bruises are often observed on toddlers, but these generally follow a specific pattern associated with minor falls and accidents. However, evidence that trauma has occurred to the child, its nature and characteristics, should never be ignored and, if possible, should be sensitively enquired about.

The importance of health visitors having knowledge of injuries associated with child abuse and neglect cannot be understated. Community nurse training and clinical supervision should ensure that nurses are familiar with the warning signs that non-accidental injury may have occurred. For example, in England and Wales, very young babies between three and five months of age are most at risk of subdural haemorrhage due to shaking injuries and these are most likely to be identified from deprived and problem households (Sanders, Cobley, Coles & Kemp, 2003). Furthermore, fractures in infants under one year of age have a high risk of being caused by abuse and neglect. Indeed, in one study of an accident and emergency department in Oxford,

UK, one in four infants presenting with fractures were identified as being non-accidental (Hoskote, Martin, Hormbrey & Burns, 2003). The younger the infant the greater the risk as the majority of identified abused infants with fractures were aged less than four months. Skeletal surveys often revealed evidence of other fractures (Hoskote et al., 2003). Thus, a missed diagnosis or identification has the potential to place a child at risk of further injury.

PREVENTION

With primary and secondary prevention, health visitors play a significant role in educating parents about their babies to reduce the chances that a child injury will occur. For example, creating a safe environment for the child to explore and educating parents about the vulnerability of children at different stages in their growth and development. It is recommended that health visitors advise parents never to shake a baby. A baby's head is too large and heavy for the neck muscles to control sufficiently. Hence, the baby's head always needs support. When shaken or roughly handled, the head can violently oscillate backwards and forwards, resulting in subdural haematoma and retinal bleeding leading to the potential for brain damage, disability and even death. Hence, shaken babies should be immediately referred to Accident and Emergency facilities for medical attention.

In addition to explaining the shaken baby syndrome to parents, it is also important to give advice on how to deal with the frustration of a persistently crying and inconsolable baby (often associated with colic). Crying often causes distress and anxiety in parents, despite the fact that it is the most common form of communication for infants. However, the parent becoming upset only frightens the baby into crying more and this vicious cycle is what needs to be prevented. The following advice can be given to parents to deal with persistent crying:

- Check the usual causes (e.g., hunger, pain (e.g., teething), wrong temperature or tired and uncomfortable).
- Give comfort to the infant through cuddling and rocking.
- Speak calmly and gently.
- Give security to the child through holding the child close to your chest so it can feel the heart beat.
- Give some time for each calming technique to work.
- As a last resort, leave the baby in a safe place, count to ten and walk away for a while to calm down and ask for immediate help from a friend or relative; check on the baby every five–ten minutes and leave again if you have to.

Similar educational approaches can contribute to the prevention of sudden infant death syndrome ('cot death') with simple advice regarding sleeping positions and temperature.

DETECTION

Tertiary prevention is offered to children and families after abuse and/or neglect has been detected. Reactive surveillance and identification of abused and neglected children leads to intervention both to stop the current maltreatment and to prevent recurrent victimisation. This is an essential service even in the presence of proactive primary and secondary preventative measures. Therefore, it is the community nurse's professional responsibility to report any suspected or actual cases of child abuse and neglect to the social services and, if necessary, refer the child to the hospital Child Protection Specialist team, who should have a designated pediatrician on call.

The relationship between injuries that occur through accidents outside the parent's control, accidents that occur as a result of a lack of supervision and trauma as a consequence of parental abuse and neglect is complex and difficult to determine. It is best seen as a dimension where, at one end, the health professional is certain that an accident outside the parent/care-giver's control has taken place and, at the other, the health professional is certain that the injury presented could only have occurred through maltreatment of the child. In between, there is the grey area about how much a lack of supervision of the child has contributed to the child's injury, for example, a child who nearly drowns by falling in a river whilst his parents were intoxicated during their picnic on a riverbank. If this failure to care is associated with neglectful behaviour or the parent being under the influence of alcohol or drugs, then there is a high risk that such injuries may reoccur in the future. Therefore, health professionals need to be aware of the factors that help identify suspected or actual child maltreatment during a doctor/nurse-patient consultation. The following questions may be helpful during consultations and medical examinations:

- Who attends with the child and what is their relationship to the child?
- What is the kind and location of the trauma/injury which has occurred (cut, fracture, burn)?
- Is this a common trauma/injury for the child's age and developmental stage?
- Is this a common location for this sort of trauma/injury?
- How does the trauma/injury look (e.g., colour, form, edges)?
- How long ago did the accident happen?

- If there is a significant delay in seeking medical attention, what is the caregiver's explanation for this?
- What is the caregiver's explanation for the cause of the trauma/injury?
- Does the story explain the type, place and location for this sort of trauma/injury?
- Who caused the trauma/injury and did other people witness the 'accident'?
- What immediate actions were taken by the parent/caregiver and were these actions adequate?
- Are there signs of old injuries/traumas?

All children and care-givers/parents attending family doctors, health clinics or being visited by community nurses in the home can be classified into a priority system of red, yellow and green for the purposes of identification of child maltreatment cases and referral. Browne and Hamilton (2003) have listed symptoms of child ill health and injury that require the doctor/nurse to consider the possibility of non-accidental injury, neglect, sexual and physical abuse when the red and yellow symptoms are present (see Table 8.1). If there is a non-matching and incongruent story from the parent to explain the child's injury (e.g., a child less than three months who has allegedly rolled over and fallen from the table to the floor), then this would raise the likelihood that non-accidental injury has occurred. Where there was unreasonable delay in seeking help after a serious injury or illness had occurred, which could not be explained by social isolation and distance from the health facility, this would raise the likelihood of abuse and neglect. Therefore, these questions are incorporated into 'good practice' history taking. Green symptoms are reassuring to the health professional in that their presence reduces the possibility of child ill health and maltreatment.

Where child abuse and neglect and/or non-accidental injury are suspected and red symptoms are present, this should lead to an emergency referral to specialists in order to determine whether child maltreatment has occurred and if immediate interventions are necessary. Where yellow symptoms are present and child abuse and neglect and/or non-accidental injury is suspected, continued assessments and home-based observation of the family are required within the next seven days. Where only green symptoms are present, standard health service provision should be followed. In the event that red or yellow symptoms co-exist with green symptoms, this indicates that there are some protective factors present and the prognosis for change and rehabilitation is more hopeful rather than poor (in the absence of green symptoms). Table 8.2 outlines potential strategies for responding to red, yellow and green symptoms.

Table 8.1 Red, yellow and green symptoms of child ill health and injury which require the doctor/nurse to consider the possibility of non-accidental injury, neglect, sexual and physical abuse

Red symptoms

- unconscious, head trauma, floppy, lethargic
- skeletal fractures (old and new)
- chest and abdomen injury
- genital and anal injury or infection
- serious burns and scalds
- severe malnutrition
- abandonment
- child frozen and hyper-vigilant

Yellow symptoms

- multiple cuts and bruises
- minor burns with inappropriate care and poor safety measures
- frequent enuresis/encupresis
- severe sleep and eating problems
- poor physical hygiene
- low height/weight for age
- developmental delay, reduced muscle tone
- little or no immunisation
- parent depressed/anxious, mentally ill, addicted
- parent discloses family violence
- parent/care-giver constantly criticises child
- child aggressive and anti-social

Green symptoms that protect children from ill-health and maltreatment

- height and weight within 'normal range'
- progressive physical and psychological development with age
- care and discipline; age appropriate and flexible
- parent* interacts and plays sensitively and consistently with the child
- parent* praises child more than criticises/rebukes
- child shows concern when separated from parent
- child smiles and seeks interaction on reunion

From Browne & Hamilton, 2003.
(* parent or substitute parent/care-giver)

CHILD PROTECTION REFERRALS

The above guidelines on detection are not meant to replace professional judgements, but may help to indicate those cases of concern. It is usually not the responsibility of the primary health care team or the community nurse to involve the police. This decision is more commonly made by social services professionals, who will instigate a joint investigation under Section 47

Table 8.2 Intervention strategies for responding to red, yellow and green symptoms where there is also a suspicion that child maltreatment has occurred

---

Red: risk of severe or life threatening injury or trauma

- *Child:*
  - Refer child urgently to hospital care and shelter
  - Specialist identifies maltreatment
  - No contact with abuser
  - Emergency legal care of child
- *Parents:*
  - Consider subsititute parental care (e.g. fostering or adoption)
  - Assess rehabilitation of non-abusive parent and child
  - Separation of violent offender
  - Criminal proceedings?

Yellow: risk of moderate to less severe maltreatment

- *Child:*
  - Family referral to social services and specialist health services
  - Child remains in family home with one or both parents (assess risk)
  - Child subject of multi-disciplinary case conference
- *Parent:*
  - Assess rehabilitation of good enough parenting
  - Closely supervise parents with daily home visits
  - Specialist psychological support and treatment, assess change

Green: no evidence of abuse or neglect

- *Child:*
  - Child safe with both parents
  - Offer health checks and refer if necessary
- *Parents:*
  - Praise and reinforce positive parenting skills
  - Review on next contact at health facility, follow up annually

---

From Browne & Hamilton, 2003.

of the Children Act 1989, if necessary. In addition to a social services referral, the primary health care team will also involve the hospital specialist child protection team (see Figure 8.1).

Especially in cases of child protection, no single professional has the knowledge or expertise to deal with this complex problem, which requires a coordinated approach from professionals in legal, medical, mental health, social work and police services.

Linking with the local social services in order to develop an agreed protocol for referral is necessary for joint working and a seamless service for families. The recommendations of the CARE programme are that these

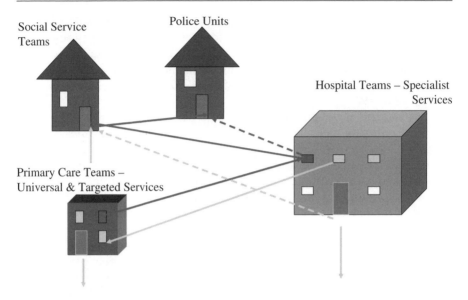

Figure 8.1 Multisector referral pathways
From Browne et al., 2005.

protocols are set up for both secondary and tertiary prevention. There should be joint agreement between primary care teams and social services to allow referrals prior to the child being maltreated and based on the health visitor identifying features that are of concern. The language used between the two services may need clarification and both organisations need to agree their identification of 'Need' and 'Significant Harm' so that community nurses can refer appropriately. Miscommunication between agencies can be a source of frustration, lost time, missed opportunities for families and can be dangerous for children. Joint protocols for referrals allow coordination of services and joint working.

From a prevention perspective, police Child Protection Units can also be very helpful when they inform health visitors of incidents of domestic violence occurring when there are children living in the household. This is because the links between spouse abuse and child maltreatment are well established but poorly recognised (Browne & Hamilton, 1999).

Drug or alcohol abuse in parents of young children is also of particular concern. These parents are often unable to attend to their infant's physical and emotional needs in a consistent and responsive manner. These infants are often physically and emotionally neglected to the point of significant harm and may be in need of care and protection outside the family unit (Iwaniec et al., 2002; Iwaniec, 2004). Therefore, health visitors should be working closely with community psychiatric nurses or mental health teams, and both should consider the implications of the parents' diagnosis and prognosis for children in the family. Indeed, adult mental health problems in parents have been implicated in some of the most serious forms of physical harm and fatal child abuse (Falkov, 1996; Reder & Duncan, 2002; Wilczynski, 1997).

However, the major problem with tertiary prevention is that significant harm may already have occurred to the child and the effectiveness of preventing further harm is relatively limited. In an English study of recurrent victimisation by Hamilton and Browne (1999), one in four children referred to police child protection units were the subject of a re-referral within a 27-month follow-up period despite social services intervention. Of those without a history of prior referrals, 57% suffered further victimisation by the same perpetrator and 43% included a new perpetrator in the follow-up period. More pessimistic findings have been provided by a Canadian study, with at least one in three children (range 33–43%) being re-referred within three years for physical abuse (MacMillan et al., 2005). Higher rates of re-referral were found for neglect (47–51%). The addition of community nurses' intervention to the standard Child Protection Agency service did not show a significant effect on re-referral (after initial abuse had occurred). This further emphasises the sometimes limited effectiveness of tertiary intervention/treatment and highlights the importance of early prediction and prevention by community nurses before problems of child abuse and neglect are identified.

9

CASE ILLUSTRATIONS OF THE CARE PACKAGE

It is often difficult to think about the application of theoretically based techniques and translate them into the clinical setting. This chapter, therefore, is designed to provide clinical illustrations of how the CARE programme has been used in a primary health care service and the types of problems it is designed to identify.

All names and details have been changed to ensure confidentiality.

CASE I. SINGLE, ISOLATED MOTHER

Mary, who was 20 years old, was pregnant with her first baby. She had been living with her boyfriend and his mother but, following an argument with her boyfriend's mother, she was thrown out of the house. Mary was living in a hostel, but was still seeing her boyfriend. She presented as a quiet, subdued young woman who wanted to improve her situation. Mary had been for interviews for jobs in local shops but had been unsuccessful in gaining employment.

Mary's midwife offered the CARE programme and she accepted the service. While discussing the items on the Index of Need, Mary revealed that her uncle (mother's brother) sexually abused her between the ages of 8 and 11 years, but her mother had not believed the allegations of sexual abuse. Mary had six other siblings and her relationship with her stepfather was very strained. She also described previous physically and sexually abusive relationships, and reported being raped on two separate occasions.

Therefore, Mary's score on the Index of Need was 12:

- Mother under the age of 21 years (1).
- Mother feels isolated with no one to turn to (1).
- Mother has serious financial problems (2).

- Mother was sexually abused as a child (2).
- Mother is single parent (3).
- Mother is having indifferent feelings about her baby (3).

Mary was in the high need category and so a plan of intervention was agreed. Although resigned to the pregnancy, she was worried that she had no money or anywhere permanent to live. Mary's self-esteem was very low and she felt rejected by everyone. She had no concept of how she would cope with the new baby and did not seem to be aware of the impact that it would make on her life. The reality of having a baby had not really entered her consciousness, as she was too concerned with her own problems and situation.

Due to Mary being able to talk about her situation with the midwife, the following services were mobilised:

- Listening visits from the midwife were to continue to provide emotional support and boost Mary's self-esteem at each contact.
- Mary was supported in her efforts to stop smoking.
- Arrangements were made for Mary to attend a supportive prenatal mother's group called 'Bumps and Babies' to share her worries, experiences and gain information and support.
- Mary was registered to start parenting preparation classes in readiness for the birth and parenthood.
- Relevant local mental health services were identified to help Mary resolve her memories about her past abuse and to manage her present abuse.
- Early referral to the health visitor was planned with full details about the case.
- A case transfer was planned within the structure of the CARE caseload so that information was not lost and services continued.

This case illustrates how the CARE programme can be used successfully by midwives, who are in a position to identify problems very early and alert the health visitors that the case will need continued services. It helps midwives move out of the role of only being focused on the physical aspects of pregnancy and birth, as well as making them alert to the responsibility of caring for a pregnant woman who is preparing for a birth in adverse emotional, social and environmental circumstances.

Women who are preoccupied with their own difficulties will not have the emotional strength to consider the needs of their unborn baby. They will not be receptive to health information being given to them about yet another stress (i.e. pregnancy and birth), unless it is provided in the context of understanding how they are feeling and coping. A mother who dreads the birth of her baby or who cannot comprehend what is going to happen cannot prepare for it or make decisions. She may not attend antenatal classes, and may not even attend for antenatal checkups. Why think about the health of a baby that is unwanted, is the result of an abusive relationship or is the reason for being made homeless? A woman in this frame of mind may be seen as unreceptive and noncompliant to services being offered, when in fact her emotional needs are so great that she does not know or even think of how to access the services. Understanding a prospective mother's feelings about her baby is crucial in enabling her to prepare, anticipate the birth and cope with her newborn.

CASE 2. FATHER'S MENTAL HEALTH PROBLEMS

Sue, who had just had her second child, was given the Index of Need by her health visitor six weeks after the birth. She completed it but nothing was disclosed and she scored under the cut off point for concern.

However, when the 3–5 month CARE visit was due, Sue suddenly phoned her health visitor to say that she was a victim of domestic violence. She said that having read the Index of Need she felt that her health visitor was the first person to contact. This new information lifted her Index of Need score to 3, which was still below the cut off. Her health visitor completed the planned visit and, after discussing the situation, agreed a plan with Sue. They agreed that Sue would

- go to her GP to discuss what had happened
- attend a local group for women who were experiencing domestic violence.

Sue was able to return to work six months after the birth. She had support from her relatives to look after her baby and continued to receive health visitor support. The father of the baby left the home and so the level of concern about the safety of the mother and child was reduced.

Two months later Sue phoned her health visitor to report that the father was back but then admitted that he had borderline schizophrenia and had stopped taking his medication. This again increased the Index of Need score.

The health visitor then liaised with the mental health team, as she was concerned for the safety of the child and the mother. She had to bridge the gap between the health visitor service and adult mental health service (AMHS) but found that issues of confidentiality in the AMHS created significant problems for her in supporting the mother and planning for the safety of the baby.

The family moved out of the area within the next few months and the CARE programme reports were transferred to the new service to ensure the continuity of protection for the baby.

This case provides an example of how the CARE programme structure enables the health visitor to revisit the Index of Need and reassess the situation in the light of new information. It may often be the case that parents may be unwilling to provide full information on the first or second contact, particularly about violence in the home or mental health problems. Going back to the Index of Need and checking on whether it has changed since the previous visit can be a prompt to some parents to think again about the information provided.

Having the Index of Need to read at home helps them understand that these issues are important to health visitors and that the health visitor may be the first person to call when they feel able to talk about their problems. Some parents are unaware that the health visitors are interested in their problems and not just about the baby. Health visitors do need to be aware that a parent may not be able to provide certain information in front of the other parent and so opportunity should always be given for parents to speak privately, if they wish to.

This case also illustrates the problems of sharing information across services. Adult health care and mental health care can have a significant impact on parents' abilities to care for their baby but issues of confidentiality can at times put a child at risk. Sharing information across child and adult services is crucial to the welfare of children.

CASE 3. SINGLE UNSUPPORTED MOTHER WITH A PREMATURE BABY

A new mother, Sarah, had just moved into a flat in the area four weeks after the birth of a 32-week gestation baby. She had already attended the GP for postnatal depression at her previous address.

When the Index of Need was introduced, the mother was very informative and communicative. She had a score of 7:

- Complication during the birth (1).
- Serious financial problems (1).
- Premature baby (2).
- Single mother (3).

Sarah had significant financial problems as her income support had stopped and her housing benefit had been disrupted. She was not registered with a GP as there was no one in the area who could take her on. In particular, Sarah was feeling lonely and unsupported, trying to cope with the uncertainties of caring for a tiny premature baby.

Sarah and the health visitor agreed a plan that included:

- Agreement with the care plan programme of visiting.
- The health visitor providing information about how to contact the Housing Department and the DSS.
- The health visitor phoning around to find a GP for the mother and baby and managing to gain agreement with one practice to take her on for three months due to their stretched services.
- Sarah completing the Edinburgh Postnatal Depression Scale to check on her level of depression one week later.
- Linking Sarah in to the pre- and postnatal support group so that she could meet new mothers and gain support.
- Linking Sarah into the Infant Massage group so that she could learn to understand and enjoy her baby.

This case demonstrated the rapid response necessary for a new mother and baby arriving in the area and the problems that a new mother can face on moving with a new baby. The health visitor was able to assess her situation rapidly and direct her to services that she required, hopefully preventing any more serious difficulties arising later as the mother failed to cope. The comprehensive and structured assessment that the CARE programme provides enables rapid and effective communication and decision-making.

CASE 4. AGGRESSIVE AND VIOLENT FATHER

Carrie was a 20-year-old mother, with two toddlers and a new baby. The health visitor's first visit for the new baby was in the home with the father present. The father, David, was considerably older than his partner but was not supportive and did little in the home to help her. The health visitor was aware of a difficult atmosphere in the house. She gave them the Index of Need to look at.

At the second visit, Carrie was alone with the children and when the Index of Need was raised, she said that she felt indifferent towards the baby. She said that her partner was not convinced that he was the father of the new baby and she did not want to discuss the Index of Need with him.

At the third visit, Carrie reported that David had violent tendencies and that he was against professionals going into the home. This created a dilemma for the health visitor because she was concerned to find out how vulnerable the children were. Carrie refused any contact with social services as she said her partner would not agree. Carrie then reported that she felt unable to leave the children alone with her partner as they might be at risk. She agreed to complete the Index of Need at this visit and had a total score of 9:

- Mother under 21 years of age (1).
- Less than 18 months between children (1).
- An adult with violent tendencies in the house (3).
- Indifferent feelings towards baby (3).
- Partner not biologically related (1) – this reflects David's belief that he is not the father because, even though it has not been proved otherwise, his view of the child is that it is not his own.

The health visitor decided that it was necessary to contact social services. Carrie agreed and the health visitor found out that David was well known to them and had previously been very aggressive to a partner and assaulted a child.

At this point, the health visitor should not have visited the home alone, but she went to find out if Carrie knew about the information from social services. She discovered that Carrie already knew the history but had not disclosed this.

The health visitor informed Carrie that she and the child were at risk and later undertook a joint visit with a social worker. There was a very hostile reception to the visit. A Child Protection Conference was held and the children were put on the Child Protection Register. David refused all help, so Carrie and the children went to the clinic for assessment, as visits to the home were too risky. A social worker and a family care worker were allocated to the family. Later, David left the home and mother and children were re-housed.

This case identifies how important it is for the health visitor to be aware of what she observes and feels on home visits, as well as what she is told by parents. However, the Index of Need presented a focus for discussion and allowed the mother to raise the issue of violence in the home. Agreement between the mother and health visitor on a plan of action was an important part of protecting the children. Some women will agree to help for the sake of the children while they will put up with violence towards themselves without admitting that it happens. The disclosure of violence in the home is critical in providing a safe environment for children to grow in.

Some health visitors may feel very unsure about when to contact social services. They may feel that this is a difficult step, particularly when one or both parents do not agree to it. However, the health visitor's prime duty is to the safety and protection of the child. She can work with parents to help them realise what services they require in order to provide a safe environment for their child, but she also must be very clear when she needs to inform them of her duty to the child. The link to social services that is possible once this issue is acknowledged helps to identify critical information that is of help in deciding on a plan of action. Sharing of information across services enables protection of children to be the priority.

CASE 5. MOTHER'S SEVERE POSTNATAL DEPRESSION

A new birth visit was planned with parents who had a new baby less than six weeks of age. The CARE Programme plan was agreed at this first visit. The parents, Jack and Sally, disclosed that the mother's previous marriage had broken up leaving two young children who also lived with them and that the mother had a history of depression after the divorce. The health visitor observed that the new partner was very supportive and involved in the care of the baby.

At the second visit, it was evident that Sally had postnatal depression, her behaviour had changed significantly and she was being violent to her partner. Their Index of Need score was 5, but they had specific needs so Sally was encouraged to go to the GP for help with her depression. Jack phoned the health visitor regularly and she visited several times as she became progressively concerned about the mother's relationship with the baby. Jack had taken paternity leave and holiday in the first couple of months after the birth and had done a lot of the care of the baby but on his return to work the mother had to take over most of the care. However, on discussion with Sally about her feelings about the baby, it was evident that she was very disengaged saying 'I don't like that baby. I didn't know how to react to it'. She felt confident with her other two children, but was detached and unresponsive to the baby.

The health visitor discussed the involvement of social services in order to gain some child care help to support the father. However, Jack was worried that the baby might be taken away and refused.

Sally's mental health and her relationship with her baby were deteriorating, so the GP and health visitor agreed a plan. A mental health community nurse visited the home twice a week in order to assess and monitor Sally's mental health, and an appointment was made for her to see an adult psychiatrist. However, an emergency call from Jack to the health visitor revealed that Sally had locked herself in the bathroom with a knife. The health visitor phoned the GP, did an immediate home visit and took two hours to persuade the mother to come out. Sally was then sectioned in order to receive appropriate mental health treatment. She made a full recovery and the health visitor was invited to the wedding.

In this case, the health visitor had a very pivotal role in supporting the father. Many men will not visit their GP and often try to cope alone. The home visit and the Index of Need allowed the father to realise that the health visitor had a wider role than just the developmental progress of the baby. He used the health visitor as his first point of contact with the services as she had visited the home and raised issues about mental and emotional health. Although ostensibly this mother had a supportive partner, her own mental health problems were critical in preventing her care appropriately for her baby. Despite the appropriate steps being taken to provide treatment for Sally's postnatal depression, a crisis did develop, but the health visitor was able to alleviate the crisis through her involvement and knowledge of the family situation. Passing over the management of parental mental health problems to other services does not mean that the health visitor no longer has a role in the care of the family. Ensuring the welfare of the children will not be the remit of the other services and so the health visitor often has a continuing role in monitoring the outcome of mental health treatment in relation to the care of the children.

CASE 6. SEVERE NEGLECT AND EMOTIONAL ABUSE

These parents, who were well known to social services, had a boy aged three years and a baby girl aged four months. They had an Index of Need score of 4:

- Financial problems (1).
- Indifferent feelings to the children (observed but not agreed by parents) (3).

The housing was poor, the hygiene very poor and there were significant financial problems, although there was a large TV and Playstation in the living room. They kept a dog that seemed to have priority over the children, as well as snakes, a rat and a tarantula. They were living in a one bedroom flat, but there was damp in the bedroom so they all moved into the lounge. They had been provided with storage boxes by social services and a skip to clear out the rubbish from the flat. They were in arrears with the council and so were not likely to be re-housed. The parents accepted no responsibility for their actions and looked after their own needs before those of the children, i.e., always had cigarettes but no milk for the baby.

Darren was not engaged with any of the support services and was volatile in mood. He had been brought up in care. Julie had poor parenting experiences herself and blocked out her childhood memories. She complained that her parents would not lend her money. She had sought out practical assistance to buy essentials for the new baby, but was seen by professionals as manipulative of services. The parents argued a lot and had left the children with a new neighbour for two weeks without thinking that they might be vulnerable. When they had left them previously with relatives, the children had returned looking chubbier and healthier.

The observation of the parenting styles and attitudes was primary in providing the health visitor with guidance about the severity of the problems. Neither parent had positive attributions about their baby, the quality of the parenting in terms of sensitivity, supportiveness, accessibility and accepting were all poor and the attachment behaviours of the baby and the three-year-old indicated insecurity. On observation, the parents were both neglectful, with poor parenting skills and poor attachment to both toddler and baby. Neither parent showed any empathy towards how the children felt.

Julie had received a lot of support and help from the health visitors, nursery nurses and midwives but there had been no significant change in her parenting style. Social services had been notified when the baby was six weeks old as she had lost weight, had repeated tummy bugs and did not feed properly. The parents had behaviour management advice in the home and from the nursery staff. However, they had been unable to use this advice and had not altered their behaviour or their complaints about the child. Julie and Darren had accepted services to keep social services at bay but had not changed their attitudes or behaviour.

The older boy was placed in a nursery for three days a week in order to protect him and give him some good social experience. He showed poor communication skills and delayed language. He was being blamed by his parents for his bad behaviour and the parents could not see how they were part of the problem.

They were re-referred to social services for a professionals meeting and a child protection case conference. The children were referred to a paediatrician due to concerns about their development. So far, no identifiable physical abuse has occurred but there is potential emotional abuse. Efforts have been made to keep the children in the family and at present there are no grounds for removal of the children. The children's names have been placed on the Child Protection Register and a core group of professionals are working with the family to improve the children's circumstances.

This family is an example where the Index of Need did not provide a high score due to lack of true information and cooperation. However, it was evident that there were significant problems and that the children's welfare was of concern. The Observational areas in the CARE programme were where the health visitor was able to record her serious concerns about parenting and attachment. The structure that these observations provide enables the health visitor to build up a cumulative picture of the child's experiences at home. The fact that on successive visits the parents' attitudes to the children do not change or modify and that the quality of parenting does not improve is valuable information for case conferences. Recording what parents say about their children and what the health visitor observes about their care during the visits within the framework of the CARE programme brings some objectivity to the professionals' opinions. The health visitor needs to be able to recognise when no change is occurring and when empowering the parents does not help the situation. Some parents need to be presented with the facts of what the professionals are observing and the effect of the family situation on the children.

CASE 7. DENIAL OF POSTNATAL DEPRESSION

Jill was a mother of three children. Observing her caring for the new baby on the first home visit, it was evident that she did not seem to enjoy interacting with him. When she changed his nappy, she did it in a rush and saw it as a task to be completed rather than an opportunity to stimulate, talk to or play with her new baby. Jill was very flippant when discussing her feelings. She was distant to the health visitor and did not seem to want to make a relationship. She said that she had no history of depression, 'I haven't got time for that.' She was given the Index of Need booklet.

On the second visit, Jill had not had time to fill in the Index of Need, but filled in the Edinburgh Postnatal Depression Scale with the health visitor and read it very carefully allowing herself time to think. When it was scored and the health visitor indicated that the score suggested that she was depressed, Jill burst into tears and said 'I've been so busy I haven't had time to think about myself. I now realise that I wasn't enjoying anything and I haven't had any support from my family or my partner.' She did not have many friends to turn to. The health visitor considered that her Index of Needs score was 4 from the information that mother had given her.

- Mother felt isolated (1).
- Indifferent feelings towards the baby (3).

However, the observation ratings revealed that Jill rarely held positive attributions towards the baby; she was rarely sensitive or supportive to him and was not accessible or accepting. On this basis, they agreed a plan of support for the mother:

- The health visitor planned a series of 'listening' visits.
- Jill was given a booklet on self help.
- The health visitor planned to see Jill's partner.
- Jill was encouraged to go to the GP for medication to manage her postnatal depression.

Following this plan, Jill received medication for her postnatal depression and made a rapid recovery. She began to cope well with being a loving mother of three.

This case again illustrates the importance of the observation ratings when the Index of Need score is low. This mother only needed a little input to help her cope, but it was timely and prevented more complex or serious problems developing.

CASE 8. USING THE INDEX OF NEED IN A GROUP FOR PREGNANT TEENAGERS

The Index of Need was discussed with a group of pregnant teenage girls as a way of raising issues that might be affecting them and to think about ways of coping with parenthood. The topics were presented to them as ideas to encourage them to think about what they could do if these things happened to them. Their initial reactions of 'nosey cow' and 'what's this got to do with us' calmed down as they began to look at the items and discuss them.

- *Complications during birth/separated from baby at birth because of poor health*

Their first reaction was 'Why should that be important?'. It provided an opportunity to discuss the importance of early attachment experiences between mother and baby after birth.

- *You or your partner under 21 years of age*

The girls were angry about this item and they could not understand why it should be important. They considered that they had equal rights to any woman to have a baby and just because they were young, it would not affect how good a mother they would be. It led to a discussion about the possible conflict between their own needs as teenagers and their own desires to go out and make relationships while they had the responsibility of looking after a baby.

- *You or your partner have a child with a physical or mental disability*

They were all scared by this topic and it provided an opportunity and an opening for them all to discuss their fears and anxieties.

- *You or your partner feel isolated with no one to turn to*

They had all felt isolated at some time in their pregnancy and through all of their bluster and bravado felt vulnerable. They raised the questions of 'Who would you trust?', 'Who would you ring?'. They were able to share suggestions about how they could all seek help and support.

- *You or your partner have serious financial problems*

Discussing finances allowed information to be given to the girls about the correct agencies to go to and the Citizens Advice Bureau and where it was.

- *You or your partner have been treated for mental illness or depression*

This topic provided an opportunity to discuss depression and some of them had already been on anti-depressants. It allowed them to think about the symptoms of postnatal depression and to recognise them. It helped them build up a sense of confidence in what they could do about it and that it can be treated once it is recognised.

- *You or your partner feel that you have a dependency on drugs or alcohol*

All the girls agreed that they had taken drugs and alcohol to excess but that they had stopped when they had found out that they were pregnant. This was because they had little money, but also because they did not want to harm their babies. They admitted that their partners had not stopped and they wondered whether this would have an influence on them after the birth. The issue of child protection was raised, as was how they could protect their babies from exposure to adults under the influence of drugs and alcohol. For example, they discussed who would care for the baby if they went out to have a drink. They were very aware of their own vulnerabilities, particularly if drugs were available. Indeed, the girls raised the issue that they would need to put their baby first, and they were all aware that the baby could be taken away if they were found to be taking drugs or putting their babies at risk. This was a very pertinent topic for them and one that exposed in particular the stresses of being a teenager and a parent.

- *You or your partner were physically or sexually abused as a child*

This topic was very relevant for several members of the group but they all only shared what they felt was appropriate within the terms of the group. They recognised the importance and sensitivity of the topic.

- *You are a single parent*

The girls said that their first reaction was to feel antagonistic because they were on their own, but then said that they realised that, 'This is why you need the support in the first place.'

- *There is an adult in the house with violent tendencies*

Many issues were raised about violence. Many of them had experienced violence from their own parents or a sibling who had rages. They thought that a baby would be too young to realise that violence was occurring and that the effect would be minimised, but they were concerned about how to keep their babies safe and discussed possible scenarios and carried out anticipatory planning.

- *You or your partner are having indifferent feelings about your baby*

They were not able to consider that they might feel indifferent toward their babies but focused on the fact that their partners were not involved.

The Index of Need proved to be a useful tool for enabling this group of girls to think about the issues that could affect them and discuss how they could manage the different scenarios. They enjoyed the group and wanted to continue even though they had been dismissive at the beginning. This illustrates how the Index of Need can be used as a tool to stimulate ideas and help prospective parents consider issues that otherwise they may be afraid to raise or may feel are irrelevant. Putting a name to the idea enables parents to express their thoughts and opinions. Even in this group of young pregnant teenagers, there were very important items that were significant in their lives; in particular dependency on drugs or alcohol and feeling isolated.

10

EVALUATION OF THE CARE PROGRAMME

Secondary Prevention involves professionals screening families and providing interventions aimed at giving special attention to high priority groups before problems arise in the parent-child relationship. As with other problems in child health and development, the risk approach to child protection can be seen as a tool for the flexible and rational distribution of resources and their maximal utilisation. Therefore, the CARE programme suggests that community nurses prioritise home visits to families based on an Index of Need.

Health and social services using this approach require the ability to identify parents and children in need of help from those characteristics (risk factors) of the child, parents, family and social environment that are associated with an increased risk of undesirable outcomes. The process, as exemplified by the CARE programme, requires resources from each local community to:

- develop methods for detecting risk factors
- train health care and social workers in these methods
- provide intervention strategies to prevent or ameliorate undesired outcomes.

The surveillance and monitoring of child health, growth and development is regarded as good practice throughout the UK and the world (Hall, 2003; WHO, 1999). The purpose of this chapter is to evaluate the assessment component of the CARE programme in terms of its predictive validity in identifying children and families in need. For the purposes of research and evaluation, the assessment procedures were related to outcome in terms of referral for suspected or actual maltreatment and the child being the subject of a child protection case conference for abuse or neglect. This outcome measure was selected in recognition of the fact that health visitors are increasingly expected to screen for and identify potential cases of child maltreatment (Robotham & Sheldrake, 2000).

Previously, a number of articles have been written on the prediction of child maltreatment (Agathonos-Georgopoulou & Browne, 1997; Altemeier et al., 1979; 1984; Ammerman, 1993; Ammerman & Herson, 1992; Leventhal, 1988; Lynch & Roberts, 1977; Starr, 1982), many of which have presented a list of characteristics common to abusing parents and to abused children (e.g., Browne & Saqi, 1988a). For example, the 'Child Abuse Potential Inventory', developed in the USA, has taken a multifaceted approach (Milner, 1986). Indeed, the CAP inventory is one of the few self-report questionnaires that has been evaluated in terms of reliability (internal consistency and temporal stability) and construct validity. However, the relevance of checklists and inventories for the prediction of child sexual abuse remains questionable, especially when the epidemiological differences between sexual and physical abuse are considered (Browne, 1994; Jason et al., 1982). Nevertheless, certain risk factors are the same, such as poor relationship with parents, step parenting, marital conflict, alcohol and drug abuse etc. (Finkelhor, 1980). Figure 10.1 gives a list of risk factors within the child and parent, the family, community and society. Hence, risk factors are identified at different levels within an ecological continuum of nested circles with all levels influencing the health and development of the child (Bronfenbrenner, 1979).

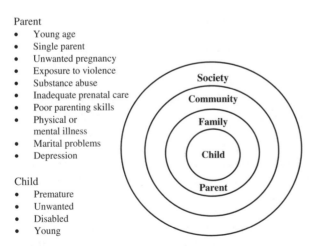

Parent
- Young age
- Single parent
- Unwanted pregnancy
- Exposure to violence
- Substance abuse
- Inadequate prenatal care
- Poor parenting skills
- Physical or mental illness
- Marital problems
- Depression

Child
- Premature
- Unwanted
- Disabled
- Young

Family
- Size
- Poverty
- Lack of social support
- Stress
- Domestic violence
- High residential mobility

Community/Society
- Lack of child protection laws
- Decreased value of children (minority, disabled)
- Social inequalities, racial and religious discrimination
- High levels and tolerance of violence (media, crime, war)
- Cultural norms (e.g., acceptance of corporal punishment)
- Absence of community services
- Poor quality health and social services
- Low social cohesion

Figure 10.1 Risk factors for child abuse and neglect
Adapted from WHO, 1999.

Various checklists and inventories draw on different combinations of these risk factors to identify families with the potential of poor outcome for the child. Community nurses have been significantly influenced in their work by such inventories, using the characteristics as 'early warning signs'. However, reviews of the relative value of these characteristics for the practical and routine monitoring of families have emphasised a need for caution because of the high number of false positives that occur (Barker, 1990; Browne, 1995bc). Nevertheless, this is inevitable when screening for a rare condition in a large population. The important feature is that community nurses should be aware that only a minority of families with a high number of risk factors will go on to abuse their children because the majority will have protective factors compensating for stressful risk factors, e.g., a good relationship between parent and child (Hamilton & Browne, 2002).

Therefore, it is not surprising that available screening tools have limited accuracy and should only be used to apply non-punitive interventions to the family. A recent systematic review (Peters & Barlow, 2003) makes this point after reviewing eight prospective studies that tested a standardised instrument to predict maltreatment around the time of birth.

EVALUATION STUDY

Information was gathered by 103 community nurses who made home visits using the CARE programme to all the families in the area. In total, 4,775 families were approached during a two-year period. This represents the total birth cohort for this area in that time. However, 310 parents refused to participate and a further 114 chose to leave the programme partway through the first six months (8.9%). Therefore, 4,351 births were screened using the Index of Need. Each infant was followed up for 13 months following birth. Within this period, 44 (1.01%) referrals were made to social services by health visitors, of which 27 infants (0.6% of total population) were referred for suspected or actual maltreatment. These figures provide a referral rate of 62 children per 10,000 in the population, which is similar to the number of children under one year of age on Child Protection Registers in England (Dept of Health, 2005b). The average age of the child at the time of the referral was 6.4 months. Table 10.1 provides the characteristics of 25 cases on which information was provided. In the other two cases, the infant was separated from the parent and/or moved out of the area and no further information was available.

The aim of the evaluation was to ascertain whether those 25 families who were referred to a child protection case conference had higher Index of Need scores and/or poor parenting ratings compared to the non-referred families, i.e., is the CARE programme effective at identifying those families at risk of harming their infants?

Table 10.1 Sample characteristics of the 25 referred families with A and B forms

Characteristic	Percentage of cases (n = 25) n (%)
Type of maltreatment referral	
Neglect	11 (44)
Physical abuse	9 (36)
Emotional abuse	4 (16)
Sexual abuse	1 (4)
Alleged perpetrator of maltreatment	
Mother only	6 (24)
Father only	7 (28)
Both parents	3 (12)
Could not be determined	9 (36)
Parental marital status	
Married	10 (40)
Cohabiting	7 (28)
Single/Separated/Divorced	8 (32)
Sex of child	
Male	12 (48)
Female	13 (52)
Child's average age at referral	6.4 months
Child's ethnic group	
White	24 (96)
Other	1 (4)

TRAINING PROCEDURES

Training procedures for the CARE programme were originally outlined in Dixon, Browne & Hamilton-Giachritsis (2005). Each health visitor involved in the CARE programme received a CARE programme Assessment Procedure Manual (see Hegarty, 2000a) together with training (Hegarty, 2000b) on the following topics:

- Partnership with parents (in-service training).
- Using the Index of Need (one-day workshop led by Professor Kevin Browne, University of Birmingham, UK).

- Case load analysis and care plans (in-service training).
- Agreeing joint referral criteria with social services (joint training initiative).
- Attachment behaviour and how to observe it (two-day workshop led by Dr. Pat Crittenden, Family Relations Institute, Miami, USA).

Therefore, expert psychologists provided three days of training on the use of risk factors and behavioural indicators to identify 'priority' families and children in need of referral to social services. This was a component of the full 10-day programme outlined above, which was organised for health visitors by Jean Hegarty, Designated Nurse for Child Protection, Southend Community Care Services (NHS) Trust. Additional inter-agency training was also organised to provide information on the CARE programme to social workers in child protection, General Practitioners, paediatricians and psychologists in the Children and Family Therapy Service.

Within the training, case studies for the identification of risk factors were presented together with video material demonstrating positive and negative parenting styles and patterns of attachment formation. In the *Assessment Procedure Manual for Health Visitors* (Hegarty, 2000a) details were given on agreed standards for interviewing the primary care-giver and responding to their comments in the context of the visit. These standardised procedures emphasised the role of the health visitor working in partnership with the mother to identify need and priority for services. To ensure these standardised procedures were used by the health visitors in a consistent and reliable way, statistical analysis was carried out on their work with families.

VISITS AND DATA COLLECTION

As outlined by Dixon, Browne and Hamilton-Giachritsis (2005), each family received a primary contact visit (new birth visit) from their health visitor. During this visit, parents were introduced to the Index of Need where they were asked to consider and identify which factors were relevant to their own family situation. Questions were phrased to access risk factors that may have been present *generally* within the family, allowing exploration of the family unit as a whole. Questions were not addressed specifically to each parent. Thus, it was not possible to separate out gender specific responses.

The Index of Need was left for both parents to discuss and complete. Preliminary feedback indicated that parents were generally responsive to this process, sometimes commenting that they had never disclosed difficulties previously because they had never been asked (Hegarty, pers. comm.).

After the introductory visit, the same health visitor visited each family when the child was 4–6 weeks of age and discussed the answers to the Index of Need with families. A total Index of Need score was calculated for each family based on the number and combination of risk factors present.

As part of the CARE programme procedures (see Dixon, Hamilton-Giachritsis & Browne, 2005; Browne, Hamilton, Hegarty & Blissett, 2000; Hamilton & Browne, 2002), health visitors also made 30-minute observations regarding the parents' attributions, perceptions and interaction with their infant, within each of the four one-hour visits. Health visitors made professional judgements about parental attributions and perceptions of infant behaviour based on discussions with the mother alone or, in a minority of cases, with both the mother and father. Additionally, at both of these visits the health visitor assessed the quality of care-giving via behavioural observation of the sensitivity, co-operation/supportiveness, accessibility and acceptance of the infant by the primary care-giver. Finally, the health visitor observed early attachment behaviour of the infant toward the primary care-giver. All of these observations were scored on a three-point scale from 'frequently' to 'rarely'.

SAMPLE ATTRITION AND RELIABILITY

As reported by Browne, Dixon and Hamilton-Giachritsis (in submission), data was provided on 4,351 families (A forms) from birth to six months. At follow-up, data was provided on 1,541 families (B forms) from seven to twelve months. This represents 35.4% of the original birth cohort. It was noted that only half the health visitors continued to submit B Forms, after they had completed the A Forms, yet they only provided data on just over one-third of the initial 4,351 sample. This may reflect smaller caseloads for the 52 health visitors that did continue to follow up families from seven to twelve months. It also indicates that the other 51 health visitors who provided nearly two-thirds of the original sample from birth to six months may have had larger caseloads. Alternatively, only those families who were considered high priority by some health visitors actually received follow-up visits. Regardless of the explanation, the evaluation indicates that large caseloads should be a consideration when implementing the CARE programme, alongside training and motivating staff to assess and evaluate need in children and their families. Ultimately, health visitors who do not perceive the value of the programme will limit its effectiveness.

It was important to determine whether those 1,541 families with A and B forms are representative of the complete screened population. A comparison with the 2,810 families with an A form only showed no significant difference for the sex of child (51% male and 49% female in both groups). Marital

Table 10.2 Prevalence of risk factors within maltreating and non-maltreating families at stages 1 and 2 of the CARE Programme Index of Need assessment

Risk factor	STAGE 1 (recorded at 4–6 weeks)		STAGE 2 (recorded at 9–12 months)	
	Referred (n = 27) n (%)	Non-referred (n = 4324) n (%)	Referred[+] (n = 25) n (%)	Non-referred[+] (n = 1516) n (%)
Complications during birth/separated from baby at birth.	3 (11.1)	482 (11.1)	3 (12.0)	140 (9.4)
Mother or partner under 21 years of age.	8 (29.6)	272 (6.3)***	8 (32.0)	56 (3.8)***
Mother or partner not biologically related to the child.	0 (0.0)	13 (0.3)	2 (8.0)	12 (0.8)*
Twins or less than 18 months between births	5 (18.5)	314 (7.3)*	5 (20.0)	120 (8.1)*
Child with physical or mental disabilities	2 (7.4)	61 (1.4)	3 (12.0)	31 (2.1)*
Feelings of isolation	7 (25.9)	115 (2.7)***	9 (36.0)	29 (2.0)***
Serious financial problems	13 (48.1)	150 (3.5)***	14 (56.0)	50 (3.4)***
Mother or partner treated for mental illness or depression	14 (51.9)	353 (8.2)***	16 (64.0)	155 (10.5)***
Dependency for drugs or alcohol	4 (14.8)	21 (0.5)***	7 (28.0)	11 (0.7)***
Mother or partner was physically and/or sexually abused as a child.	9 (33.3)	126 (2.9)***	8 (32.0)	51 (3.4)***
Infant seriously ill, premature or weighed under 2.5 kg at birth	3 (11.1)	240 (5.6)	1 (4.0)	66 (4.5)
Single parent	9 (33.3)	272 (6.3)***	9 (36.0)	90 (6.1)***
Adult in the household with violent tendencies	7 (25.9)	42 (1.0)***	7 (28.0)	15 (1.0)***
Mother or partner feeling indifferent about their baby	2 (7.4)	48 (1.1)*	3 (12.0)	9 (0.6)***

* = p < 0.05, ** = p < 0.01, *** p < 0.001 Fishers Exact tests; [+] valid percentages used.

status of the families also showed no significant differences between the two groups. Overall, the mothers were recorded as 6% single, 25% cohabiting, 68% married and 1% separated, divorced or widowed. These records showed consistency with the information recorded on the Index of Need form, which also showed single parents to represent 6% of the non-referred population at 4–6 weeks (Form A) and 9–12 months (Form B). Other risk factors on the Index of Need also showed no significant differences for families with A and B forms (stage 2) compared to families with A forms only (stage 1), regardless of whether they were referred or not (see Table 10.2).

The mean Index of Need score at birth for those families with an A form only was 0.97 compared to 1.02 for those families who had both Forms A and B completed. Again, this was not significantly different. In relation to the health visitors' observations at both 4–6 weeks and 3–5 months, the mean ratings also showed no significant differences between the groups for the following:

- Parental attributions about the infant.
- Parental perceptions of infant behaviour.
- Quality of parenting.
- Infant attachment formation.

Overall, the sample of 1,541 families with data across all four visits was representative of the original 4,351 cohort on which data around the time of birth was provided. This suggests that health visitors were **not** visiting what they perceived to be high priority families for the third and fourth visits. Therefore, the continuation of visits was more likely to be related to caseloads and health visitor motivation.

FINDINGS

Index of Need

Statistical comparisons of the Index of Need (Form A) at 4–6 weeks after the infant's birth, between 27 referred cases for child maltreatment and 4,324 non-referred families, showed significant differences on 10 of the 14 risk factors (see Table 10.2). Additionally, a comparison of average scores found that referred families had a significantly higher Index of Need score at 4–6 weeks (mean = 6.11; SD = 3.534) than non-referred families (mean = 0.95; SD = 1.695), (t_{26} = 7.578, p < 0.001).

Statistical comparisons of the Index of Need (Form B) at 9–12 months, between 25 referred cases for child maltreatment and 1,516 non-referred families, showed significant differences on 12 of the 14 risk factors (see Table 10.2). A comparison of average Index of Need scores obtained by referred (mean = 7.08; SD = 3.651) and non-referred families (mean = 0.93; SD = 1.696) was also significantly different (t_{24} = 8.41, p < 0.001), with the referred families again showing a higher score.

Table 10.3a Prevalence of positive parenting styles shown by referred and non-referred parent families at stage 1 of the CARE Programme

Positive parenting styles	STAGE 1 (N = 4351)			
	4–6 weeks		3–5 months	
	Maltreating (n = 27)	Non-maltreating (n = 4324)	Maltreating (n = 27)	Non-maltreating (n = 4324)
Positive attributions and realistic perceptions				
Mother's attributions regarding infant	21	4123***	23	4123**
Father's attributions regarding infant	12	3769**	11	3718***
Mother's perceptions of infant	21	4118***	23	4144**
Father's perceptions of infant	12	3757**	13	3778*
Positive quality of care giving behaviours				
Sensitivity	23	4144**	22	4141***
Supportiveness/ co-operativeness	20	4134***	21	4144***
Accessibility	21	4108***	21	4123***
Acceptance	22	4107**	22	4136***

* = p < 0.05, ** = p < 0.01, *** p < 0.001.

PARENTING STYLES

The frequency of positive parenting styles conducted by both maltreating and non-maltreating parent families at stages 1 and 2 of the CARE programme are displayed in Table 10.3ab. Parenting styles were recorded at two different time intervals within each stage, at 4–6 weeks and 3–5 months of stage 1 (Form A) and 6–8 and 9–12 months of stage 2 (Form B). Fishers Exact Probability Test demonstrated that non-maltreating families were signifi-

Table 10.3b Prevalence of positive parenting styles shown by referred and non-referred parent families at stage 2 of the CARE Programme

Positive parenting styles	STAGE 2 (N = 1 541)			
	6–8 months		9–12 months	
	Maltreating (n = 25)	Non-maltreating (n = 1 516)	Maltreating (n = 25)	Non-maltreating (n = 1516)
Positive attributions and realistic perceptions				
Mother's attributions regarding infant	17	1 463***	18	1 447***
Father's attributions regarding infant	7	1 361***	6	1 344***
Mother's perceptions of infant	16	1 464***	18	1 466***
Father's perceptions of infant	6	1 357***	6	1 356***
Positive quality of care giving behaviours				
Sensitivity	18	1 462***	17	1 467***
Supportiveness/ co-operativeness	19	1 462***	17	1 472***
Accessibility	19	1 459***	18	1 466***
Acceptance	16	1 454***	17	1 458***

* = p < 0.05, ** = p < 0.01, *** = p < 0.001.

cantly more likely to be positive in their attributions and perceptions of their child, and in the quality of their parenting, across each time interval of both stages 1 and 2 of the CARE programme.

INFANT ATTACHMENT BEHAVIOUR

Table 10.4 depicts the frequencies of attachment behaviours displayed by maltreated and non-maltreated infants, across the four time intervals within Stages 1 and 2 of the CARE programme. Fishers Exact Probability Test found

Table 10.4 Prevalence of infant attachment behaviours displayed by referred and non-referred infants at Stages 1 and 2 of the CARE Programme

Infant attachment behaviours	Maltreating	Non-maltreating
Stage 1 (4–6 weeks)	**(n = 27)**	**(n = 4324)**
Infant smiles at care-giver	21	3565
Infant quietens when picked up by care-giver	21	4125**
Infant responds to care-giver's face	21	4091*
Infant eye contact and scanning	21	4131**
Infant settles in care-giver's arms	23	4143
Stage 1 (3–5 months)		
Infant turns head to follow care-giver	22	4134***
Infant responds to care-giver's voice with pleasure	20	4087***
Infant imitates speaking to care-giver	20	3970**
Infant shows preference for being held by care-giver	21	4000**
Stage 2 (6–8 months)	**(n = 25)**	**(n = 1516)**
Infant shows a preference for the primary care-giver	19	1362*
Infant demonstrates some distress when left by the primary care-giver	11	1120**
Infant is confident to explore	15	1214*
Infant is relaxed, 'comforted' when held by the primary care-giver	17	1463***
Stage 2 (9–12 months)		
Insecure attachment with care-giver	2	22

* = $p < 0.05$, ** = $p < 0.01$.

that non-maltreated infants displayed a significantly greater frequency of the majority of infant attachment behaviours. However, significant differences did not emerge between groups in terms of 'Infant smiles at care-giver' (Fishers Exact = 1.000, $p > 0.05$) and 'Infant settles in care-giver's arms' (Fishers Exact = 0.075, $p > 0.05$) at 4–6 weeks after the child's birth.

At stage 2, all attachment behaviours significantly differentiated between groups but an insecure attachment patten was rare in both maltreated and non-maltreated infants according to health visitor classifications.

Predictive Validity

The problem for health visitors is that they are only likely to come across six in every 1,000 families where the child is being maltreated by their parents. This comparatively rare condition makes it difficult for any screening instrument to be highly sensitive and accurate.

Nevertheless, a statistical analysis was performed to see how well the Index of Need discriminated between the 27 referred cases and the 4,324 non-referred families using the data from Form A. Using the weightings and overall scores, the Index of Need is sensitive to 70.4% (19) of the 27 referred cases for child protection but misses 29.6% (8) of the 27 referred cases as they do not have a high score. With reference to the 4,324 non-referred families, the Index of Need correctly specified 96.4% (4167) as not in need, but incorrectly labelled 3.6% (157) as being in need due to their high score. Overall, 96.2% of families were correctly classified into their respective referred and non-referred groups (see Figure 10.2). A similar discrimination was found for the 1,541 families using Index of Need data from Form B.

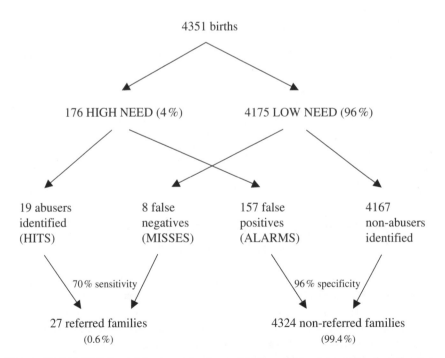

Figure 10.2 CARE Programme evaluation of Index of Need completed at the time of birth (n = 4,351) as determined by discriminant function analysis

To further distinguish the 19 'hits' from the 157 'false alarms' in the 176 high need families identified, information on parental behaviour is necessary. This information may also help to pick out the eight 'missed' cases in the 4,175 low need families, although of course this will be much more difficult.

IMPLICATIONS FOR PRACTICAL APPLICATION OF THE INDEX OF NEED

The evaluation of the CARE programme shows that a score of 5 or more is the best cut-off score on the Index of Need. This would pick up a high number of families who will actually go on to be referred while limiting the number of false alarms (i.e., seen as high risk but not referred).

An Index of Need score of 5 or more will be sensitive to over two-thirds (70%) of child protection referrals with a 4% false alarm rate. By comparison, a cut-off score of 6 or more would yield less than half (only 45%) of the child protection referrals, although the false alarms would be reduced to 2.6% of the families not likely to be referred. Alternatively, a cut-off point of 4 or more would identify three-quarters (75%) of the child protection referrals but at a cost of 8.4% of non-referred families being incorrectly classified as 'false alarms' in high need.

It is recommended, therefore, based on an evaluation with families in Essex that those families who score 5 or more should be placed in priority for further home visits and community nurse support. Parents in these 'high priority families' should be counselled and helped to find ways to reduce the risk factors present. This may involve referrals to other community services and agencies. Nevertheless, health and social service professionals should keep in mind that only one in every nine families in need (19 from 176 Essex families) are likely to be referred for child protection issues from the 4% of the newborn population identified as belonging to 'high priority families' (see Figure 10.2).

INDICATORS OF PARENTING BEHAVIOUR AND THEIR CONSISTENCY

Those families with a high Index of Need score of 5 or more were significantly more likely to have parents with negative attributions and perceptions toward their baby and poor quality of parenting in comparison to other families. These parenting behaviour indicators were observed to be consistent in families and correlate at 4–6 weeks, 3–5 months, 6–8 months and 9–12 months. Consequently, the developmental indicators of infant attachment were also observed to be consistently less good in 'high priority families' and correlate at 4–6 weeks, 3–5 months and 6–8 months. Therefore, those families with a high Index of Need score and poor parenting should be deemed to be most in need as their child is likely to have the poorest outcome. These families require urgent referral to family centres and community support groups as well as close monitoring and support from health and social service professionals. In the rare event of a health visitor observing parents from a 'low priority family' (low index of need score) with negative attributions and perceptions toward the baby and poor quality of parenting, this family should be counselled and offered advice on positive parenting. Such a case may represent one of the two per 1,000 low priority families that are referred for child protection difficulties (see Figure 10.2).

THE IMPORTANCE OF PROGRAMME EVALUATION

The Index of Need cut-off score of 5 or more, determined from an evaluation of Essex families offers a guide for other areas but may not be the most effective cut-off point for other populations. This is due to geographical variations in the performance of risk factors. Where a risk factor is common in a particular population (e.g., economic problems such as unemployment) then the predictive value of this established risk factor will be limited. Hence, the weighted score for this factor in a rural locality may not be as effective in an urban locality.

The fact that the Index of Need distinguishes families likely to have poorer outcomes for their children across localities confirms the fact that the list of risk factors and indicators of poor parenting is robust in their association with poor outcome at both a national and international level. It is the relative performance, and hence weightings, of these factors which vary from population to population. For example, the Essex community health professionals first applied a cut-off score of 6 or more based on research from Surrey families (Browne and Saqi, 1988; Browne and Herbert, 1997). As can be seen above this is not the best balance between being sensitive to referral cases and limiting false alarms (or false positives). An advantage of the higher cut-off score is that the targeted service cost less as fewer families were identified as 'High Priority' (3% of the newborn Essex population) but less than half of potential child protection referral families were picked up in Essex within the first 6 weeks after birth.

Only after evaluating the presentation of risk factors and parenting indicators in referred cases compared to non-referred families (for a specific area/ population) can the most cost-effective cut-off point be determined. At least one to two years postnatal follow-up is required to classify screened families based on outcome (e.g., child protection referral) after the CARE programme has been implemented.

In the case of Essex, an expensive targeted service sensitive to three-quarters of potential child protection referrals would require interventions with 8% of the newborn population (with a cut-off score of 4 or more). The recommended compromise is to prevent problems in at least two-thirds of potential child protection referrals from birth at a cost of targeted services to 4% of the newborn population (with a cut-off score of 5 or more). Nevertheless, this compromise may be considered unethical in that more children may be harmed by parents who have been missed (false negatives). Only by programme evaluation in each specific population/locality can informed decisions be made. The importance of costing in evaluation into the programme cannot be understated.

11

CONCLUSION –
THE COST-EFFECTIVENESS
OF COMMUNITY NURSE
HOME VISITING

Governments have a difficult challenge balancing the needs and rights of children with the needs and rights of parents, which can create tensions for policy makers when all of these needs are in conflict or competing. According to Henricson and Bainham (2005), a balance is best achieved by policy makers who provide primary preventative strategies and universal support to children and their families together with committing resources to transparent and multi-disciplinary child protection systems that focus on intervention and rehabilitation.

Over the past decade, the importance of early interventions with parenting has been shown to be the most effective way of promoting the optimal development of children and preventing child abuse and neglect in families (Browne, Hanks, Stratton & Hamilton, 2002). This research evidence has influenced government policies towards identifying the needs of children, the parents' capacity to meet those needs and the social and environmental factors that impinge on the parents' capacity as a Framework for the Assessment of Children and their Families (Dept of Health et al., 2000). This has led to an emphasis on providing services to those in need at an early stage (Dept of Health, 1999; Home Office, 1998). Indeed, the CARE Programme became a part of the Sure Start initiative (Dept of Education and Employment, 1999), as it was recognised as a good practice model for early intervention.

The CARE Programme provides a strategy and structure to help implement the recommendations of the Children Act (2004), which focuses on early intervention with children and their families through the development of preventative services, such as positive parenting programmes, new children's centres and the involvement of schools in community-based initiatives. This 'public health' approach has a much broader remit for children's services as it integrates child care and protection with the monitoring and welfare of child health and development. This places children with disabilities centre stage with those who require protection or specialised health care. Children with special needs are assessed along with all other children as part of the routine primary health care. These needs assessments are best carried out using community home visits by health visitors.

The design of the CARE programme has many of the features of successful home visiting programmes as identified by Guterman (1997):

- Early identification and/or screening of families referred through a universalistic services system (i.e., parents identified via the health service in the antenatal period).
- Initiation of supportive services during pregnancy or shortly after birth.
- Voluntary participation.
- In-home service provision.
- Case management support.
- Provision of parenting education, guidance and support.
- Frequent visits over an extended period of time (i.e., over six months).
- Programme delivered by trained professionals.
- Integration of the service within existing services.

In terms of child protection, the effectiveness of the public health approach, with its shift from treatment to prevention through community home visits, is yet to be determined. Some question whether this may be at the expense of strengthening front-line child protection (Bell, 2004). However, the difficulties and failings of rescuing children from child maltreatment, rather than preventing it in the first place were clearly implicated in the Victoria Climbié report. Furthermore, the community-based public health approach to primary and secondary prevention of child maltreatment appears to be much less expensive than tertiary intervention, which only offers help after abuse and neglect has occurred.

There are two issues with intervening after maltreatment occurs. First, the child has already suffered harm and is at increased risk of further maltreatment. Research has shown that approximately one-quarter (24%) of children referred to police child protection units in the UK are re-referred within 27 months (Hamilton & Browne, 1999). In the USA, rates of re-referral after initial contact with child protection agencies range between 8% and 13% for the same child in a four year follow-up (Fryer & Miyoshi, 1994). When any child in the family is counted as the re-referral though, the rate rises to 50% with a five-year follow-up and as high as 85% of families in a ten-year follow-up (DePanfilis & Zuravin, 1998). Secondly, it has been stated that the 'true' cost of child maltreatment needs to account for the medical care for victims, mental health provision for victims, legal costs for public child care, criminal justice and prosecution costs, treatment of offenders, social work provision and specialist education. Thus, this was estimated in 1996 to be a total economic cost of £735 million per year in the UK (€ 1.1 billion) and $12,410 million (€ 12.4 billion) per year in the USA (WHO, 1999).

COSTS AND BENEFITS OF PRIMARY AND SECONDARY PREVENTION

Given the high costs associated with the consequences of child maltreatment, it is useful to consider this against the costs of implementing primary and/or secondary forms of prevention. The Triple P Positive Parenting Programme (Sanders, 1999) has been estimated to cost only €26 per 2–12 year old child to implement (i.e., the cost for 572,701 children was €14,805,000), with research showing that Triple P can reduce prevalence of childhood behaviour problems by 26% (Mihalopoulos et al., in submission). Using the total economic cost for the UK in 1996 (WHO, 1999), this gives a potential saving of €286,650,000 (Mihalopoulos et al., in submission).

A weekly community nurse home-visiting programme targeted to disadvantaged first time mothers, who were under 21 years of age, single parents and with serious financial problems, has been evaluated in the USA. Olds et al. (1993) showed that the cost of providing home visiting per family was $1,582 US dollars. However, this intervention by a community nurse saved $1,762 US dollars in the first two years of the child's life. Hence, there was an overall net saving (dividend) of $180 US dollars per family (in the 1980s). There was a 56% saving in family aid, 26% in food stamps, 11% in medical aid and a 3% decrease in child protection cases. There was also a 5% increase in income tax received from an increase in maternal part-time employment resulting from the professional advice given. Given this evidence, it is surprising to observe a reduction in the community nursing services in the UK. In fact, it could be argued that it would be more cost-effective to double the number of community nurses available to families. Nevertheless, it should be recognised that the training of general practitioners, community psychiatric nurses, health visitors and midwives requires a greater focus on child protection. Without this re-focusing, there will be a reliance on tertiary prevention at greater financial and human cost.

SERVICE DELIVERY

In the UK, community nurse home-visits occur for all mothers with newborns as a universal primary care service. Research in Surrey (Browne &

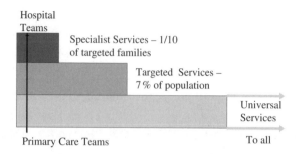

Figure 11.1 The build up of health services that children and their families receive
From Browne et al., 2005.

Saqi, 1988) showed that only 7% of those families visited required targeted services and only one in 10 of these high priority families were later subject to a child protection conference and received specialist services (see Figure 11.1). It is important to understand that targeted and specialist services occur at an additional health cost and do not replace universal primary care. Services are built up to match the needs of the child and the family so that targeted services are added to universal primary care services already received by the family. For those few families that require specialist services, these services are also offered in addition to the continuation of targeted and universal primary care services. Therefore, support services for children and their families are built up in layers as depicted in Figure 11.1.

Programmes that include routine community nurse home-visits to families in a defined population have been shown to be more effective at preventing physical child abuse and neglect than those programmes where community nurses only visit families using a screening measure (Guterman, 1999). This demonstrates the importance of maintaining a standard service to all families even when screening measures are used to identify families who require more intensive support.

EFFECTIVENESS OF COMMUNITY NURSE HOME VISITS

The effectiveness of community nurse visitation programmes has been the subject of three systematic reviews (Elkan et al., 2000; Hahn et al., 2003; MacMillan et al., 2000) in the past five years. The most comprehensive review of 102 studies by Elkan et al. (2000), evaluating 86 programmes and 174 assessments, found an association between home visiting programmes and the following factors:

- Improvements in parenting skills and the quality of home environment.
- Amelioration of several child behavioural problems.
- Improved intellectual development among children especially children with a low birth weight or failure to thrive.
- A reduction in the frequency of unintentional injury and a reduction in the prevalence of home hazards.
- Improvements in the detection and management of postnatal depression.
- Enhancement of quality of social support to mothers.
- Improved rates of breastfeeding.

In addition, Hahn (2003) reviewed 51 assessments from a much smaller sample of studies meeting their more specific inclusion criteria and found that home visitation programmes in the US:

- Reduced incidents of child abuse and neglect where other forms of domestic violence are absent.
- Were more effective than paraprofessionals.
- Produced cost savings on health care.

Macmillan et al. (2000), with a review of 15 home visitation programmes in the USA, found greater effectiveness in reducing child abuse and neglect for first time mothers with low income. Furthermore, MacLeod and Nelson (2000) noted that home visiting programmes with fewer visits and shorter durations (i.e., less than six months) are less effective.

However, the above findings are to be treated with caution as not all home visitation programmes consistently produce the same results. This is because of the inconsistency in the methods used to target families, which showed great variation across the studies reviewed. Some of these variations are a consequence of cultural and social circumstances of the families studied. For example, there is no universal health visiting service in North America where most of the evaluated home visiting programmes are located. By contrast, the small number of European studies (mainly in the UK and the Netherlands) have, as a foundation, universal primary care services to all families prior to any targeting/selection process (e.g., Brocklehurst, Barlow, Kirkpatrick, Davis & Stewart-Brown, 2004; Browne et al., 2000; Grietens, Geeraert & Hellinckx, 2004). Therefore, a combined review of home visitation programmes is dominated by the North American model, which may not perform in the same way, or to the same extent in a European context. Therefore, it is essential to carry out a scientifically controlled evaluation (random controlled trial) on a community nurse home visitation programme in the UK.

GUIDELINES AND TRAINING

In relation to the prevention of family violence, child maltreatment and its later consequences, the Department of Health in England (1999) have published guidelines on the responsibility of community nurses to recognise and refer families according to the following recommendations.

- Set up a communication system with social work services, primary care teams and family practitioners about current concerns.
- Regularly review caseloads with colleagues to ensure all the information about the child and the family is available and recorded.
- Set up a system of formal notification and participate in case conferences.
- Collect and report information about missing families and no access visits where there is cause for concern as a child has not been seen or assessed.
- Ensure effective communication with the midwife involved with the family especially during the handover of the responsibility approximately 10 days after birth (continuity of care through prenatal health visiting is preferable).
- Prioritise the time necessary to assist in prevention work with families.
- Establish appropriate systems of record keeping and reporting in relation to assessment and intervention.

The necessity of these guidelines for health visitors has been demonstrated by a UK study carried out in South London by Gilardi (1991). This study showed that 97% of health visitors had been directly involved in at least one case of child abuse and neglect and over 70% in five or more cases. In 42% of child protection cases, the health visitor was first to suspect abuse.

These guidelines are useful for training health professionals and, in particular persuading general practitioners to think more deeply about child protection issues. Due to a number of factors, only 16% of General Practitioners regard attendance at child protection conferences as essential (Simpson et al., 1994). In a review of 200 consecutive child protection conferences, there was no primary care team input (attendance or written report) by either the GP or the health visitors in 32% of cases and only 10.5% of child protection conferences were attended by GPs (op cit).

Ideas for engaging GPs in child protection training have been offered by Hendry (1997), but she acknowledges that despite increased efforts and postgraduate educational allowance, GP attendance at child protection events is disappointing. Bannon et al. (1999) suggest a fresh approach using primary health care teams as a focus for the development of training in this area. GPs themselves have identified a desire for training in how to promote child welfare in instances of child maltreatment, whilst protecting themselves from criticism or litigation. There is no legal mandate to report British cases of child abuse and neglect to the police and social services, but there is a clear expectation that doctors 'must refer these concerns to the statutory agencies' (Department of Health, British Medical Association, Conference of Medical Royal Colleges, 1994).

Nevertheless, any involvement of health professionals in child protection work must be seen in the broader context of multi-disciplinary networking and referral processes.

CONCLUSION

Given the research evidence on the cost-effectiveness of community nurse home-visits, it is surprising to observe a reduction in the community nursing services in the UK and other parts of Europe. In fact, it could be argued that it would be more cost-effective to double the number of community nurses available to families. Nevertheless, it should be recognised that the training of general practitioners, community psychiatric nurses, health visitors and midwives requires a greater focus on child protection. Without this re-focusing, there will be a reliance on tertiary prevention at greater financial and human cost.

Appendix 1

'LOOKING AT YOUR NEEDS' BOOKLET FOR MIDWIVES

Using the
CARE Programme
(Child Assessment, Rating and Evaluation)
'Looking at your needs'

In partnership
with

The
**Public Health
Midwife**

Being pregnant –

- Can bring about many changes in our emotions based on our own upbringing and present life experiences.

Becoming a parent –

- Sometimes encourages us to remember past experiences from our own childhood that we may have managed to forget.
- Some of these memories are pleasant to recall and help us decide what sort of parent we would like to be ourselves. Other memories may upset or alarm us such as remembering how we suffered physical or sexual abuse at the hand of an adult entrusted to care for us.
- Other problems such as housing problems, financial pressures, relationship difficulties and isolation may also prevent us from enjoying our parenting experience, simply through worry.

A Community Health Approach to the Assessment of Infants and Their Parents: The CARE Programme. By K. Browne, J. Douglas, C. Hamilton-Giachritsis and J. Hegarty.
Copyright © 2006   John Wiley & Sons, Ltd.

But what about you as an individual?

We are all unique as individual human beings.
Life events such as becoming parents or increasing the size of our families
can bring about many changes in our emotions based on our upbringing
and present life experiences.

So what can we do?

The health care team can work in partnership with you via our midwife to
look at your needs.

What do we mean by that?

Well, let's face facts – we cannot wave a magic wand and make all hurts and
problems disappear for you, we cannot add to the family income or provide
new housing.

But we can . . .

- During your pregnancy provide support, guidance, information and
  develop your confidence in your parenting skills by regular contact with
  your Public Health Midwife and others in the health care team.
- Provide health education advice throughout your pregnancy.
- Ensure that you know how to make use of all the services that may be
  beneficial to your own personal needs.
- Listen to you and help you receive the help that would most benefit
  you.

So how does a parent decide what their needs are?

Years of research have been undertaken in Britain and the rest of the world
in order to identify the circumstances that cause most stress to parents
during pregnancy. There are factors which time and time again suggest help
will be required in order for adults to enjoy being parents and their infants
receive the love, care and attention that is their right.

So what is the next step?

- We will invite you to answer some questions and award yourself a
  score.
- First of all don't worry if you feel unable to answer a question – that can
  be very understandable.
- Remember, you can always go back to the list and think again or even
  change your mind about something.

- Next, discuss your needs with your Public Health Midwife – tell her the score you have decided is the right one for you.

What will the Public Health Midwife do?

- She will look at your needs.
- She will work with you to get the help you seem to require based on your answers and what you wish to say about them.

Remember

- We believe you and your family are the most important reason for our professional existence.
- We also wish to work within the spirit of the 1989 Children Act where it states we have a duty to work in partnership with parents, and that children have the right to be protected and have resources provided for them if they are deemed 'in need'.
- We also believe that you have responsibilities as parents and that by working in partnership with you, we can assist you to fulfil and achieve those responsibilities as parents especially in times of stress.
- We believe we can only provide appropriate services by asking you to take full partnership with our services.
- We invite you to look at your needs as prospective parents, check out your feelings about yourself, your partner and your unborn baby.

How do you as would-be parents decide what your needs are?

- There are factors that suggest help will be required in order for adults to enjoy being parents and their children to receive the love, care and attention that is their right.

We now invite your to look at your needs.

- First of all, either on your own or as a couple, or with your Midwife, take stock of your present situation

Check out your feelings about

- you
- your partner
- your unborn baby
- your life

What sort of things are you saying to yourself?
What sort of things is your partner saying?

Do you wish to talk about the sort of things you hear yourself saying in your mind?

- Next read the following list of researched factors carefully and decide what applies to you and your family – give yourself a score.

FACTORS	SCORE
You had (a) serious complications during birth, and/or (b) were separated from your baby after the birth because of your poor health	1
You or your partner are under 21 years of age	1
You or your partner are not biologically related to the child	1
You had twins or there is less than 18 months between births of your newborn and previous child	1
You have a child with physical or mental disabilities	1
You or your partner feel isolated with no one to turn to	1
You have serious financial problems	2
You have been treated for mental illness or depression	2
You feel that you have a dependency on drugs or alcohol	2
You or your partner were physically or sexually abused as a child	2
Your infant is (a) seriously ill (b) premature (c) weighed under 2.5 kgs at birth	2
You are a single parent	3
There is an adult in the house with violent tendencies	3
You or your partner are having indifferent feelings about your baby	3
	—
TOTAL	

What next?

- If you have a score of 5 or over, it is likely you will require further services. Your midwife will discuss all of the options with you.

Should you have further questions, or simply wish to talk over any thoughts or feelings you have about the questionnaire before your next appointment, contact:

Name

Designation

Number

Or

Name

Designation

Number

Together we can plan the services or action that you feel would benefit you and your family.

Meanwhile,

**Kind regards
from your midwife and the
Health Care Team**

Appendix 2

'LOOKING AT YOUR NEEDS' BOOKLET FOR HEALTH VISITORS

Using the
CARE Programme
(Child Assessment, Rating and Evaluation)

'Looking at your needs'

In partnership
with

The
Health Visiting
Service

Dear Parent (s)

Your health visitor extends her warmest congratulations to you on the birth of your baby.

What is a health visitor?

Your health visitor is a community nurse who concentrates upon preventative care. All health visitors are registered general nurses. Many of them are also midwives or have other relevant qualifications. Extra training has been undertaken to qualify as a health visitor. NHS Trusts employ health visitors to call on families in their homes, especially where there are new babies and

A Community Health Approach to the Assessment of Infants and Their Parents: The CARE Programme. By K. Browne, J. Douglas, C. Hamilton-Giachritsis and J. Hegarty.
Copyright © 2006 John Wiley & Sons, Ltd.

small children. The service is mainly educational and supportive, aiming to improve community health and empowering parents by helping them to feel confident in rearing small children.

Health visitors are professionally qualified and experienced in the normal development of infants and children; therefore, they can offer developmental assessments to children and identify deviations from normal at an early stage. They are interested in the health and welfare of all family members, which includes mid-life as well as the elderly. They have counselling skills and can be supportive to you in times of family stress.

When a baby is born

Life changes in many ways. Most of the issues relating to change are covered at antenatal classes by midwives and health visitors and through the excellent health educational publications that most parents receive. All of this information is generally considered to be useful as a 'blanket' response to providing the population with helpful advice.

But what about you as an individual?

We are all unique as individual human beings.
Life events such as becoming parents or increasing the size of our families can bring about many changes in our emotions based on our upbringing and present life experiences.

Did you know?

- That having a baby sometimes encourages us to remember past experiences from our own childhood that we may have managed to forget.

What sort of memories?

- Some of these memories are pleasant to recall and help us decide what sort of parent we would like to be ourselves. Other memories may upset or alarm us such as remembering how we suffered physical or sexual abuse at the hand of an adult entrusted to care for us.

Feelings about present circumstances

- Other problems such as housing problems, financial pressures, relationship difficulties and isolation may also prevent us from enjoying our parenting experience, simply through worry.

So what can we do?

The health care team can work in partnership with you via your health visitor to look at your needs.

What do we mean by that?

Well, let's face facts – we cannot wave a magic wand and make all hurts and problems disappear for you, we cannot add to the family income or provide new housing.

But we can. . . .

- During the first year of your baby's life, provide you with support, guidance, information and develop your confidence in your own parenting abilities by regular contact with the health visitor and child health clinic.
- Provide health education advice for family fitness and wholeness.
- Ensure you know how to make use of all the services that may be beneficial to your personal needs and requirements.
- Provide advice clinics on sleep, toddler behaviour and special needs support groups.
- Put you in touch with nursery and child minding facilities, mother and toddler groups, postnatal support or postnatal depression groups, social services facilities, voluntary groups support and counselling services.
- Assist you to improve your own care and support by offering appropriate help, and in some cases in a befriending role, to acquire the help you need from other agencies.

So how does a parent decide what their needs are?

Years of research have been undertaken in Britain and the rest of the world in order to identify the circumstances that cause most stress to parents during pregnancy and early parenting. There are factors which time and again suggest help will be required in order for adults to enjoy being parents and their infants receive the love, care and attention that is their right.

So what is the next step?

- We will invite you to answer some questions and award yourself a score.
- First of all don't worry if you feel unable to answer a question – that can be very understandable.

- Remember, you can always go back to the list and think again or even change your mind about something.
- Next, discuss your needs with your health visitor – tell her the score you have decided is the right one for you.

What will the health visitor do?

- She will look at your needs.
- She will work with you to get the help you seem to require based on your answers and what you want to say about them.

Will the health visitor assess my needs as well?

Yes. Please do not worry and think you have been given all of the responsibility. Your health visitor will be making her own assessment along with you. She will share her observation with you and together you can discuss and finally decide on the course of action you require.

What if I change my mind?

- You have the right to change your mind, after all, you may remember something that you originally forgot or felt unable to talk about.
- Your circumstances may change during the year and you may wish to alter something in your list of needs.
- Your health visitor may have altered her initial assessment as well, due to your altered circumstances. All of this is understandable and we will accommodate any new ideas you may have.

Remind me again – why do I need to take part in this?

- We believe you and your family are the most important reason for our professional existence.
- We also wish to work within the spirit of the 1989 Children Act where it states we have a duty to work in partnership with parents, and that children have the right to be protected and have resources provided for them if they are deemed 'in need'.
- We also believe that you have responsibilities as parents and that by working in partnership with you, we can assist you to fulfil and achieve those responsibilities as parents especially in times of stress.
- We believe that most parents know what is best for their own situation, therefore, we value your own assessment as well as our own professional judgements.

- We believe we can only provide appropriate services by asking you to take full partnership with our services.
- We invite you to look at your need as prospective parents, check out your feelings about yourself, your partner and your unborn baby.

We now invite you to look at your needs.

- First of all, either on your own or as a couple, or with your Midwife, take stock of your present situation

Check out your feelings about

- you
- your partner
- your unborn baby
- your life

What sort of things are you saying to yourself?
What sort of things is your partner saying?
Do you wish to talk about the sort of things you hear yourself saying in your mind?

- Next read the following list of researched factors carefully and decide what applies to you and your family – give yourself a score.

FACTORS	SCORE
You had (a) serious complications during birth, and/or (b) were separated from your baby after the birth because of your poor health	1
You or your partner are under 21 years of age	1
You or your partner are not biologically related to the child	1
You had twins or there is less than 18 months between births of your newborn and previous child	1
You have a child with physical or mental disabilities	1
You or your partner feel isolated with no one to turn to	1
You have serious financial problems	2
You have been treated for mental illness or depression	2
You feel that you have a dependency on drugs or alcohol	2
You or your partner were physically or sexually abused as a child	2
Your infant is (a) seriously ill (b) premature (c) weighed under 2.5 kgs at birth	2
You are a single parent	3
There is an adult in the house with violent tendencies	3
You or your partner are having indifferent feelings about your baby	3
TOTAL	

What next?

- If you have a score of 5 or over, it is likely you will require further services. Your health visitor will discuss all of the options with you.

Should you have further questions, or simply wish to talk over any thoughts or feelings you have about the questionnaire before your next appointment, contact:

Name_____

Designation_____

Number_____

Or

Name_____

Designation_____

Number_____

Together we can plan the services or action that you feel would benefit you and your family.

Meanwhile,

**Kind regards
from your
Health Visiting Service**

Appendix 3

FORM A
BIRTH TO FIVE MONTHS

THE *CARE* PROGRAMME

(CHILD ASSESSMENT RATING AND EVALUATION)

BROWNE – HAMILTON – WARE 1995

CARE PROGRAMME

H.V. Name ....

Baby's D.O.B. ....

Sex ....

Patient I.D. 1st letter of name .... 1st 2 letters of s'name ....

1. Occupation before birth of child

		Mother	Father
0	Not known	❑	❑
1	Professional	❑	❑
2	Managerial	❑	❑
3	Skilled non manual	❑	❑
4	Skilled manual	❑	❑
5	Unskilled non manual	❑	❑
6	Unskilled manual	❑	❑
7	Armed forces	❑	❑
8	Unemployed/ retired	❑	❑
9	Student	❑	❑
10	House person	❑	❑

2. Ethnic Origin

....

3. Marital status

1 ❑ Single
2 ❑ Living together
3 ❑ Married
4 ❑ Separated
5 ❑ Divorced
6 ❑ Widowed

4. Relationship to the child

	Mother	Father
Natural parent	❑	❑
Step parent	❑	❑
Cohabitee	❑	❑
Adoptive/foster parents	❑	❑
Non-resident partner	❑	❑

5. Score on Edinburgh Postnatal Depression Scale (4–6 weeks) ❑

INDEX OF NEED AT 4–6 WEEKS

H.V. Name .... This index of need is completed
in consultation with parents (unless
parents refuse – please indicate below)

Baby's D.O.B. ....

Sex .... The index score should be based
on the parents' self report and
the health visitor's professional
opinion of known factors

Patient I.D. **Please tick area**

❏ ❏ ❏

1st letter of name .... ❏ ❏ ❏

❏ ❏ ❏

1st 2 letters s'name .... ❏ ❏ ❏

Please circle alphabetical key	Factors (If father is absent seek mother's opinion)	Please circle relevant score
A	Complications during birth/separated from baby at birth because of poor health.	1
B	You or your partner under 21 years of age.	1
C	You or your partner are not biologically related to the child.	1
D	Twins or less than 18 months between births of newborn and previous child.	1
E	You or your partner have a child with physical or mental disabilities.	1
F	You or your partner feel isolated with no one to turn to.	1
G	You or your partner have serious financial problems.	2
H	You or your partner have been treated for mental illness or depression.	2
I	You or your partner feel that you have a dependency drugs or alcohol.	2
J	You or your partner were physically or sexually abused as a child.	2
K	Your infant is (a) seriously ill (b) premature (c) weighed under 2.5 kgs at birth.	2
L	You are a single parent	3
M	There is an adult in the house with violent tendencies.	3
N	You or your partner are having indifferent feelings about your baby.	3

Parent/s refusal ....
(Please tick)

Unborn babies who are case conferenced
require another form to be completed.

TOTAL INDEX SCORE

....

OBSERVING ATTACHMENTS & ATTRIBUTIONS

H.V. Name   ....   Patient I.D.....................

Baby's D.O.B.   ....   1st letter of name ....

Sex   ....   1st 2 letters s'name.......

Please tick if father/father figure present.

❏ Yes
❏ No

---

1. Attributions: (How the parent(s) speak about and to the infant)

	Frequently positive	Occasionally positive	Rarely positive
Mother	❏	❏	❏
Father	❏	❏	❏

(if father is absent seek mother's advice)

---

2. How parents perceive infant behaviour

	Mostly realistic	Occasionally realistic	Rarely realistic
Mother	❏	❏	❏
Father	❏	❏	❏

(if father is absent seek mother's advice)

---

3. Quality of parenting: Primary care-giver to infant

	Frequently	Occasionally	Rarely
1. Sensitive	❏	❏	❏
2. Supportive/co-operative	❏	❏	❏
3. Accessible	❏	❏	❏
4. Accepting	❏	❏	❏

ATTACHMENT   Specify primary care-giver   ❏ Mother   ❏ Father   ❏ Other

---

4. Infant to primary care-giver

	Frequently	Occasionally	Rarely
1. Smiles at care-giver	❏	❏	❏
2. Quietens when picked up by care-giver	❏	❏	❏
3. Responds to care-giver's voice	❏	❏	❏
4. Eye contact and scans care-giver's face	❏	❏	❏
5. Settles in care-giver's arms	❏	❏	❏

OBSERVING ATTACHMENTS AND ATTRIBUTIONS

AGED 3–5 MONTHS

H.V. Name   ....

Please tick if father/ ❏ Yes ❏ No
father figure present.

Baby's D.O.B.   ....
Sex   ....

1. Attributions: (How the parent(s) speak about and to the infant)

	Frequently Positive	Occasionally positive	Rarely positive
Mother	❏	❏	❏
Father	❏	❏	❏

Patient I.D.:
1st letter of name   ....
1st 2 letters s'name   ....

2. How parents perceive infant behaviour

	Mostly realistic	Occasionally realistic	Rarely realistic
Mother	❏	❏	❏
Father	❏	❏	❏

(If father is absent seek mother's opinion)

3. Quality of parenting: Primary care-giver to infant

	Frequently	Occasionally	Rarely
1. Sensitive	❏	❏	❏
2. Supportive/co-operative	❏	❏	❏
3. Accessible	❏	❏	❏
4. Accepting	❏	❏	❏

ATTACHMENT   Specify primary care-giver   ❏ Mother   ❏ Father   ❏ Other

4. Development of attachment behaviour 3–5 months:

	Frequently	Occasionally	Rarely
1. Turns head to follow care-giver's movements	❏	❏	❏
2. Responds to care-giver's voice with pleasure – windmill movements of arms/kicking legs	❏	❏	❏
3. Imitates 'speaking' to care-giver by moving lips in response to care-giver	❏	❏	❏
4. Shows preference for being held by care-giver by settling and quieting	❏	❏	❏

Appendix 4

FORM B
SIX MONTHS TO ONE YEAR

THE *CARE* PROGRAMME

(CHILD ASSESSMENT RATING AND EVALUATION)

BROWNE – HAMILTON – WARE 1995

CARE PROGRAMME

H.V. Name   ....

Baby's D.O.B. ....

Sex   ....

Patient I.D.:   1st letter of name   ....

                1st two letters of s'name ....

Marital status

1 ❑ Single   2 ❑ Living together 3 ❑ Married   4 ❑ Separated
5 ❑ Divorced 6 ❑ Widowed

Changes in family circumstances

			Specify
Change in marital status	Yes ❑	No ❑	....
Change in partner	Yes ❑	No ❑	....
Change in occupation	Yes ❑	No ❑	....

* If new partner
A. Sex   Male ❑ Female ❑   (please tick)
B. Ethnic group   ....
C. Occupation   ....
D. Relationship to child(ren) ....

OBSERVING ATTACHMENTS AND OTHER ATTRIBUTIONS

AGED 6–8 MONTHS

H.V. Name   ....   Please tick if father/father
Baby's D.O.B.   ....   figure present.
Sex   ....
Patient I.D.:   ❑ Yes
1st letter of name ....   ❑ No
1st 2 letters s'name ....

---

1. **Attributions: (How the parent(s) speak about and to the infant)**

	Frequently positive	Occasionally positive	Rarely positive
Mother	❑	❑	❑
Father	❑	❑	❑

(If father is absent seek mother's opinion)

---

2. **How the parents perceive infant behaviour**

	Mostly realistic	Occasionally realistic	Rarely realistic
Mother	❑	❑	❑
Father	❑	❑	❑

---

3. **Quality of parenting: Primary care-giver to infant.**

	Frequently	Occasionally	Rarely
1. Sensitive	❑	❑	❑
2. Supportive/co-operative	❑	❑	❑
3. Accessible	❑	❑	❑
4. Accepting	❑	❑	❑

Attachment Specify primary care-giver ❑ Mother ❑ Father ❑ Other

---

4. **Attachment in the making 7 to 8 months**

	Frequently	Occasionally	Rarely
1. Shows preference for a primary care-giver	❑	❑	❑
2. Demonstrates some distress when left by primary care-giver	❑	❑	❑
3. Confident to explore – crawls away from primary care-giver, turns around to look at primary care-giver	❑	❑	❑
4. Relaxed, 'comforted' when held by primary care-giver	❑	❑	❑

INDEX OF NEED AT 12 MONTHS

H.V. Name   ....   This index of need is completed in consultation with parents (unless parents refuse – please indicate below)

Baby's D.O.B.   ....   The index score should be based on the parents' self report and the health visitor's professional opinion of known factors

Sex   ....   Compare form 'B' with form 'A' to detect any changes over the past year

Patient I.D.:   **Please tick area**

1st letter of name   ....

1st 2 letters s'name   ....

Please circle alphabetical key	Factors (if father is absent seek mother's opinion)	Please circle relevant score
A	Complications during birth/separated from baby at birth because of poor health	1
B	You or your partner under 21 years of age	1
C	You or your partner are not biologically related to child	1
D	Twins or less than 18 months between births of new born and previous child	1
E	You or your partner have a child with physical or mental disabilities	1
F	You or your partner feel isolated with no-one to turn to	1
G	You or your partner have serious financial problems	2
H	You or your partner have been treated for mental illness or depression	2
I	You or your partner feel that you have a dependency on drugs or alcohol	2
J	You or your partner were physically or sexually abused as a child	2
K	Your infant is (a) seriously ill (b) premature (c) weighed under 2.5 kgs at birth	2
L	You are a single parent	3
M	There is an adult in the house with violent tendencies	3
N	You or your partner are having indifferent feelings about your baby	3

Parent/s refusal
(Please tick)

Unborn babies who are case conferenced
require another form to be completed.

TOTAL INDEX
SCORE

....

OBSERVING ATTACHMENTS AND OTHER ATTRIBUTIONS

AGED 9 MONTHS–1 YEAR

H.V. Name .... Patient I.D.: Please tick if father/
Baby's D.O.B. .... 1st letter of name .... father figure present.
Sex .... 1st 2 letters s'name .... ❑ Yes
    ❑ No

---

1. Attributions: (How the parent(s) speak about and to the infant)

	Frequently positive	Occasionally positive	Rarely positive
Mother	❑	❑	❑
Father	❑	❑	❑

(If father is absent seek mother's opinion)

---

2. How the parents perceive infant behaviour

	Mostly realistic	Occasionally realistic	Rarely realistic
Mother	❑	❑	❑
Father	❑	❑	❑

(If father is absent seek mother's opinion)

---

3. Quality of parenting: Primary care-giver to infant.

	Frequently	Occasionally	Rarely
1. Sensitive	❑	❑	❑
2. Supportive/co-operative	❑	❑	❑
3. Accessible	❑	❑	❑
4. Accepting	❑	❑	❑

ATTACHMENT   Specify primary care-giver   ❑ Mother   ❑ Father   ❑ Other

Indicate which type of attachment is applicable by ticking the appropriate box

1. Avoidant attachment (insecure) Tends not to seek interaction with care-giver and does not become distressed when separated from care-giver. On reunion with care-giver, often resists physical contact.

2. Independent attachment (secure) Often seeks interaction, but not especially physical contact. Is rarely distressed on separation. On reunion greets care-giver by smiling and reaching out.

3. Dependent attachment (secure) Actively seeks physical contact and interacts with care-giver. On reunion greets care-giver by smiling and reaching out.

4. Ambivalent attachment (insecure) Low levels of play, lack of interaction and obvious anxiety with strangers with intense distress on separation. On reunion they may continue to cry and mix contact seeking behaviour with active resistance to the care-giver's approaches.

HEALTH VISITORS COMPLETION STUDY

Observational guide

	Excellent 1	Good 2	Adequate 3	Poor 4	Inadequate 5
Safety Child awareness safety standards within the home (e.g.) poisons or medicines locked away; training to avoid accidents, dangerous situations; child not left alone	❑	❑	❑	❑	❑
Food Parents feeding child?	❑	❑	❑	❑	❑
Shelter Standards of accommodation (e.g., a warm, dry bed; some privacy; a place for his or her property; a place to play?)	❑	❑	❑	❑	❑
Cleanliness Hygiene and attention to hair and skin care?	❑	❑	❑	❑	❑
Appearance Appropriate clothing (warm and tidy)?	❑	❑	❑	❑	❑

Adapted from Herbert (1991) with permission.

Sensitive responsiveness to the infant:

(Base your ratings for categories below on a representative of observation)

Does the care-giver or parent:	Always	Most of the time	Sometimes	Never
	1	2	3	4
Responds promptly to the infant's needs?	❏	❏	❏	❏

Infants have very limited abilities to appreciate the consequences of their own behaviour; an interval of only 3 seconds disrupts the learning of 6-month-old infants. Where the adult takes appreciably longer to answer the infant's signals there will be no opportunity to learn that his or her behaviour can influence the behaviour of other people.

Respond appropriately to his or her needs?	❏	❏	❏	❏

This means the ability to recognise the particular 'messages' the infant is trying to communicate, and to interpret and react to them correctly.

Respond consistently?	❏	❏	❏	❏

A child's environment must be predictable; he or she must be able to learn that his or her behaviour will produce particular consequences under particular conditions.

Interact smoothly and sensitively with the infant?	❏	❏	❏	❏

Parents can mesh their interactions with infants in a manner that is facilitative and pleasurable as opposed to intrusive and disruptive.

Adapted from Herbert (1991) with permission.

Overall rating of psychological care

Rate the quality of psychological care provided for the child based on observations and interview data

	Excellent	Good	Adequate	Poor	Inadequate
Affection	❑	❑	❑	❑	❑

This includes physical contact, admiration, touching, holding, comforting, making allowances, being tender, showing concern, communicating, monitoring the child's activities.

Security	❑	❑	❑	❑	❑

This means continuity of care, a predictable environment, consistent controls, settled patterns of care and daily routines, fair and understandable rules, harmonious family relationships.

Guidance and control	❑	❑	❑	❑	❑

Discipline appropriate to the child's stage of development, providing a model to emulate, imitate, indicating limits, insisting on concern for others.

Independence	❑	❑	❑	❑	❑

Making opportunities for him or her to do more for themselves; make decisions, first about small things, but gradually about larger matters.

Stimulation (including new experiences)	❑	❑	❑	❑	❑

Stimulation by encouraging curiosity and exploratory behaviour, by praising and encouraging, by responding to questions and play, and by promoting training and educational opportunities.

Adapted from Herbert (1991) with permission.

HEALTH VISITORS COMPLETION SUMMARY

Please indicate any referrals which you indicated during the first year following your assessments and CARE Programme observations.

Health
❏ GP
❏ C.M.O.
❏ Paediatrician
❏ Psychiatrist
❏ C.P.N.
❏ Other (please specify)
....

Social Services
❏ Children in need
❏ Child protection
❏ Nursery placement

On the Child Protection Register
❏ Yes
❏ No

Health Visiting Service
❏ S.A.F.E. Group (Post-natal depression)
❏ H.A.L.O. Group (Behaviour-coping)
❏ Sleep Clinic (Infant sleep problems)
❏ Home is where we start from (Specialist parenting group)
❏ H.E.L.P. Group (Health visitors counselling project)

Voluntary Groups
❏ Network Family Group
❏ Home Start
❏ Mother and Toddler
❏ Counselling ....
  (please specify)
....
❏ Other ....
  (please specify)
....

Specify the number of home visits undertaken during the first year of the infant's life

Primary Prevention: Routine surveillance   . . . .
Secondary Prevention: Supplementary support   . . . .

CASE MANAGEMENT BEYOND ONE YEAR

Indicate which option you have planned for the child(ren)'s care

❏ Routine surveillance   or   ❏ Prolonged active management
If prolonged active management has been indicated please specify the factors that you perceive as relevant in deeming the child(ren) as 'in need' or 'of concern' on your caseload.

....
....

Appendix 5

FORM C
THE CARE PROGRAMME
(CHILD ASSESSMENT RATING
AND EVALUATION)

BROWNE – HAMILTON – WARE 1995

THIS FORM MUST BE COMPLETED FOR EVERY CHILD AT RISK
OF 'SIGNIFICANT HARM' OR DEEMED TO BE IN NEED OR
REQUIRING PROTECTION

**IF MORE THAN ONE CHILD IS REFERRED AT THE SAME TIME,
THE FORM SHOULD BE COMPLETED ON THE YOUNGEST CHILD**

A Community Health Approach to the Assessment of Infants and Their Parents: The CARE Programme. By K. Browne, J. Douglas, C. Hamilton-Giachritsis and J. Hegarty.
Copyright © 2006   John Wiley & Sons, Ltd.

INDEX OF NEED

H.V. Name .... This index of need is completed in consultation
Patient's D.O.B. .... with parents (unless parents refuse – please
indicate below)

Sex ....

Patient I.D.   The index score should be based on the
1st letter of name   parent's self report and the health visitor's
1st 2 letters s'name   professional opinion of known factors

<u>Please complete the following checklist,
re-checking the family characteristics
at the time of referral.</u>

Please circle alphabetical key	Factors (if father is absent seek mother's opinion)	Please circle relevant score
A	Complications during birth/separated from baby at birth because of poor health	1
B	You or partner under 21 years of age	1
C	You or your partner are not biologically related to child	1
D	Twins or less than 18 mths between births of newborn & previous children	1
E	You or your partner have a child with physical or mental disabilities	1
F	You or your partner feel isolated with no one to turn to	1
G	You or your partner have serious financial problems	2
H	You or your partner have been treated for mental illness or depression	2
I	You or your partner feel that you have a dependency on drugs or alcohol	2
J	You or your partner were physically or sexually abused as a child	2
K	Your infant is (a) seriously ill (b) premature (c) weighed under 2.5 kgs at birth	2
L	You are a single parent	3
M	There is an adult in the house with violent tendencies	3
N	You or your partner are having indifferent feelings about your baby	3

Parent/s refusal . . . . . .
(Please tick)

TOTAL INDEX
SCORE

....

Family and Siblings

	Parental/Guardian Situation	
H.V. Name	Two Natural Parents	❑
Baby's D.O.B.	Mother Alone	❑
Sex	Mother/Father Substitute	❑
Patient I.D.	Father Alone	❑
1st letter of 1st name	Father/Mother Substitute	❑
1st 2 letters S'name	Relative	❑

If more than 1 child is
referred at the same time,
the form should be completed
on the youngest

Foster Parent ❑
Adoptive Parent ❑
L.A. Care ❑
Other (Please Specify) ......

Siblings

D.O.B.	Gender	Relationship to child (e.g. half/full/step)	Known abused/ suspected/not	Currently of concern for referral
Eldest first				
1.	....	....	....	Yes/no
2.	....	....	....	Yes/no
3.	....	....	....	Yes/no
4.	....	....	....	Yes/no
5.	....	....	....	Yes/no

If sibling(s) have been or are suspected of being abused answer:

Type of Abuse	Perpetrator	Age when abused
1.	....	....
2.	....	....
3.	....	....
4.	....	....
5.	....	....

If siblings are currently on the Child Protection Register

Date of Conference   ❑ ❑   ❑ ❑   ❑ ❑ ❑ ❑

Category of Registration
(please tick)

Mixed ❑
Physical ❑
Emotional ❑
Neglect ❑
Sexual ❑

Have siblings been registered or case conferenced in the past? ❑ Yes ❑ No

CARE Programme

(Child protection)

H.V. Name ....
Baby's D.O.B. ....
Sex ....
Patient I.D.
1st letter of 1st name ....
1st 2 letters S'name ....

Referral Details

Date of referral ....
Reason for referral ....

---

1. IN NEED (Section 17 Children Act)

    Impairment of health   A) Physical
                                          B) Emotional

    Impairment of development   A) Physical
                                          B) Emotional
                                          C) Intellectual
                                          D) Social

2. PROTECTION (Section 47 Children Act)

    Ill Treatment   A) Physical abuse
                                          B) Neglect
                                          C) Emotional abuse
                                          D) Sexual abuse
                                          E) Mixed

Are you referring one child	Yes ❏	No ❏
Are you referring all of the children	Yes ❏	No ❏

CARE Programme

(Child protection)

H.V. Name ....
Baby's D.O.B. ....
Sex ....
Patient I.D.
1st letter of 1st name ....
1st 2 letters S'name ....

Reason for Referral (Physical)

Nature of child's injury/reason for referral (please tick whichever were present)

PHYSICAL   ❏ No Physical Injury   ❏ Child's report
           ❏ Bruising   ❏ Others report
           ❏ Lacerations
           ❏ Fractures
           ❏ Haematoma
           ❏ Burns/scalds
           ❏ Poisoning
           ❏ Illness Induction
           ❏ Breathing or Choking Problems

Anatomical area of child's physical injuries at the time of referral

Head   ❏ Scalp   Trunk ❏ Chest   Face ❏ Mouth
       ❏ Skull   ❏ Abdomen   ❏ Eyes
       ❏ Ears   ❏ Back   ❏ Cheeks
       ❏ Cerebral

Limbs ❏ Arms   Genitals ❏ Labia   ❏ Not Applicable
       ❏ Hands   ❏ Vulva
       ❏ Legs   ❏ Testes
       ❏ Feet   ❏ Penis
                             ❏ Anus

Degree of most serious injury   ❏ Minor
                                                        ❏ Moderate
                                                        ❏ Severe
                                                        ❏ Fatal

See attached definitions sheet

Reason for Referral (continued)

H.V. Name
Patient's D.O.B.
Sex
Patient I.D.
1st letter of name
1st 2 letters of s'name

❑ Child's report
❑ Others report

SEXUAL: ❑ Sexualised behaviour
               ❑ Repeated urinary infections
               ❑ Vaginal discharge (STD)
               ❑ Pregnancy (under age)
               ❑ Vaginal bleeding in pre-pubescent child
               ❑ Anal/vaginal injuries

NEGLECT: ❑ Failure to thrive
                 (in absence of organic illness)
               ❑ Inappropriately clothed for weather conditions
               ❑ Poor hygiene – skin, hair, personal hygiene
                 Severe nappy rash/skin lesions
               ❑ Parents not taking advice
               ❑ OTHER (Please specify) ....
               ....
               ....

EMOTIONAL: ❑ Persistent negative attitudes towards child
               ❑ Persistent denigration, harsh discipline
                 and over control
               ❑ Terrorising
               ❑ Leave alone
               ❑ Confining the child in frightening situations
               ❑ OTHER (Please specify)

SEVERITY OF ABUSE: ❑ Less severe
                       ❑ Moderately severe
                       ❑ More Severe
                       ❑ Life threatening

See attached definitions

ALLEGED PERPETRATOR

H.V. Name
Patient's D.O.B.
Sex
Patient I.D.
1st letter of name
1st 2 letters of s'name

❑Mother
❑Father
❑Stepmother/Co-hab
❑Stepfather/Co-hab
❑Foster/Adoptive Mother
❑Foster/Adoptive Father
❑Siblings
❑Brother   D.O.B. ....
❑Sister   D.O.B. ....
❑Extended Family – Male   Specify ....
❑Extended Family – Female   Specify ....
❑Family Friend
❑Person in Trust   Specify ....
❑Another Child(ren)
❑Another Adolescent(s)
❑Stranger
❑Other   Specify ....

Was the perpetrator a known Schedule 1 offender?   ❑ Yes
                                                        ❑ No

Did the perpetrator have a history of ill treatment or
neglect of other children?   ❑ Yes
                                                        ❑ No

Referral Outcome

H.V. Name _____
Baby's D.O.B. _____
Sex _____
Patient I.D.
1st letter of 1st name _____
1st 2 letters S'name _____

1. **Investigation** ❑ (a) Run checks
   ❑ (b) Strategy Meeting
   ❑ (c) Joint investigation
   ❑ (d) No further action
   ❑ (e) Child Protection
          Conference

2. **Legal Action**
   ❑ (a) Emergency Protection Order
   ❑ (b) Child Assessment Order
   ❑ (c) Interim Care order
   ❑ (d) Full Care Order
   ❑ (e) Police Protection Order

3. **Accommodation**

   ❑ (a) Remains with parent(s)

   ❑ (b) Placed with relatives

   ❑ (c) Foster Care (Short term)

   ❑ (d) Foster Care (Long term)

   ❑ (e) Adoption

4. **Contact**

   ❑ (a) Mother supervised
   ❑   Mother unsupervised
   ❑   Withheld
   ❑   No contact from choice

   ❑ (b) Father supervised
   ❑   Father unsupervised
   ❑   Withheld
   ❑   No contact from choice

5. **Contact With Significant Others:**

	Siblings	Contact with siblings
		Contact withheld
State if child has supportive contact with siblings, grandparents or other family members	Grandparents	Maternal
		Contact withheld
		Paternal
		Contact withheld
Other family member _____		Contact withheld

CHILD PROTECTION CONFERENCE

H.V. Name
Patient's D.O.B.
Sex
Patient I.D.
1st letter of name
1st 2 letters of s'name

Was a Child Protection Conference convened?   Yes ❑   No ❑

If yes: Date of Conference ....
Category: ❑ Initial
                     ❑ Review

Outcome:

(a) Registration ❑

Category:	Likely	Actual
Physical Abuse	....	....
Sexual Abuse	....	....
Emotional Abuse	....	....
Neglect	....	....

In some cases more than one Category of Registration may be appropriate. However, multiple abuse registrations should not be used to cover all eventualities.
Please tick categories according to conference outcome.

Date of Next Conference: ....

(b) Not registered ❑
(c) De-registered ❑

Decision Making: If children were not registered was it:
                      Majority decision? ....
                      Casting vote by Chairperson? ....
                      Do you agree with the decision?   Yes ❑ No ❑

Category: a) The original factors which led to abuse no longer apply ❑
             b) The child has remained at home but the risk of abuse has reduced due to work with the family ❑
             c) The child has been placed away from home and the risk is no longer present ❑
             d) The abusing adult is no longer a member of the household and the child has no further contact ❑
             e) The risk assessment has revealed that registration is no longer required ❑
             f) The child is no longer a child in the eyes of the law ❑

LEGAL INTERVENTION

H.V. Name
Patient's D.O.B.
Sex
Patient I.D.
1st letter of name
1st 2 letters of s'name

Are social services planning:

        a)   ❏ To request legal advice?

        b)   ❏ To seek a Child Protection Order?

        c)   ❏ To seek an interim Care Order?

        d)   ❏ To seek a full Care Order?

        e)   ❏ To seek a Supervision Order?

        f)   ❏ To seek an Assessment Order?

        g)   ❏ To convene a Child Care Planning Meeting?

        h)   ❏ You are unsure of social services' intentions.
Please expand ....
....
....
....

Re-activated Case

H.V. Name _____
Baby's D.O.B. _____
Sex _____
Patient I.D.
1st letter of 1st name _____
1st 2 letters S'name _____

<u>Has this child been previously case conferenced?</u> ❏ Yes ❏ No

If yes, were they registered?   ❏ Yes ❏ No

Category of registration	Likely	Actual
Physical		
Sexual		
Emotional		
Neglect		

Date of previous registration   _____

Date of removal from the register   _____

Category of de-registration   <u>Please specify</u>

....
....
....
....

Length of time between incidents _____

<u>Severity</u>   More severe than present incident
                                        Equal severity
                                          Less severe

<u>Number of referrals made</u>   A) The Child(ren)
                                    B) The Family

DEFINITION SHEET ON

SEVERITY OF MALTREATMENT
(From Browne and Herbert, 1997)

LESS SEVERE

Minor incidents of an occasional nature with little or no long-term damage
– either physical, sexual or psychological.

- Physical e.g.: Injuries confined in area and limited to superficial tissues,
  including cases of light scratch marks, small slight bruising, minute
  burns and small welts.
- Sexual e.g.: Inappropriate sexual touching, invitations and/or
  exhibitionism.
- Emotional e.g.: Occasional verbal assaults, denegration, humiliation,
  scapegoating, confusing atmosphere.
- Neglect e.g.: Occasional withholding of love and affection, weight parallel
  to or slightly below third centile with no organic cause.

MODERATELY SEVERE

More frequent incidents and/or of a more serious nature, but unlikely to be
life-threatening or have such potentially long-term effects.

- Physical e.g.: Surface injuries of an extensive or more serious nature and
  small subcutaneous injuries, including cases of extensive bruising, large
  welts, lacerations, small haematomas and minor burns.
- Sexual e.g.: Non-penetrative sexual interaction of an indecent or inappropriate nature; such as fondling, masturbation and digital
  penetration.
- Emotional e.g.: Frequent verbal assaults, denegration and humiliation,
  occasional rejection.
- Neglect e.g.: Frequent withholding of love and affection, non-organic
  failure to gain weight.

VERY SEVERE

Ongoing or very frequent maltreatment and/or less frequent incidents with
potentially very severe physical or psychological harm.

- Physical e.g.: All long and deep tissue injuries and broken bones (including fractures, dislocations, subdural haematomas, serious burns and
  damage to internal organs).

- <u>Sexual</u> e.g.: Sexual interaction involving attempted or actual oral, anal or vaginal penetration.
- <u>Emotional</u> e.g.: Frequent rejection, occasional withholding of food and drink, enforced isolation and restriction of movement.
- <u>Neglect</u> e.g.: Frequent unavailability of parent, guardian or spouse, non-organic failure to thrive.

LIFE THREATENING

Long-term or severe psychological and physical harm that results in life threatening situations (including perpetrators failing to seek help in time or victims harming themselves).

- <u>Physical</u>: Deliberate or persistent injuries which have the potential of victim death or near death.
- <u>Sexual</u>: Incest, coerced or forced penetration over a prolonged period.
- <u>Emotional</u>: Persistent rejection, failure to nurture, frequent withholding of food and drink, enforced isolation and restriction of movement.
- <u>Neglect</u>: Persistent unavailability of parent, guardian or spouse, non-organic failure to maintain weight.

REFERENCES

Abidin, R. (1990) *Manual of the Parenting Stress Index (PSI)* (3rd edn). Charlottesville, VA, University of Virginia, Pediatric Psychology Press.

Adcock, M. & White, R. (1985) *Good-enough Parenting: a Framework for Assessment.* London, British Agencies for Adoption and Fostering.

Adcock, M. & White, R. (1998) *Good-enough Parenting: a Framework for Assessment* (2nd edn). London, British Agencies for Adoption and Fostering.

Agathonos-Georgopoulou, H. & Browne, K.D. (1997) The prediction of child maltreatment in Greek families. *Child Abuse and Neglect* **21(8)**: 721–735.

Ainsworth, M.D.S. (1977) Infant development and mother-infant interaction among Ganda and American families. In P.H. Leiderman, S.R. Tulkin & A. Rosenfeld (eds), *Culture and Infancy: Variations in the Human Experience* (pp. 119–150). NY, Academic Press Inc.

Ainsworth, M.D.S., Blehar, M.C., Waters, E. & Wall, S. (1978) *Patterns of Attachment: a Psychological Study of the Strange Situation.* Hillsdale, NJ, Erlbaum.

Altemeier, W.A., Vietze, P., Sherrod, K., Sandler, H., Falsey, S. & O'Connor, S. (1979) Prediction of child maltreatment during pregnancy. *Journal of the American Academy of Child Psychiatry* **18**: 205–218.

Ammerman, R.T. (1993) Physical abuse and neglect. In T. Ollendick & M. Hersen (eds), *Handbook of Child and Adolescent Assessment* (pp. 439–454). Boston, Allyn and Bacon.

Ammerman, R.T. & Hersen, M. (1990) *Treatment of Family Violence.* New York, John Wiley & Sons, Inc.

Ammerman, R.T. & Hersen, M. (1992) *Assessment of Family Violence: a Clinical and Legal Sourcebook.* New York, John Wiley & Sons, Inc.

Anisfeld, E., Casper, V., Nozyce, M. & Cunningham, N. (1990) Does infant carrying promote attachment? An experimental study of the effects of increased physical contact on the development of attachment. *Child Development* **61**: 1617–1627.

Balbernie, R. (2001) Circuits and circumstances: The neurobiological consequences of early relationship experiences and how they shape later behaviour. *Journal of Child Psychotherapy* **27**: 237–255.

Bamrah, J.S., Freeman, H.L. & Goldberg, D.P. (1991) Epidemiology of schizophrenia in Salford, 1974–84: changes in an urban community over ten years. *British Journal of Psychiatry* **159**: 802–810.

Bannon, M.J., Carter, Y.H., Barwell, F. & Hicks, C. (1999) Perceptions held by General Practitioners in England regarding their training needs in child abuse and neglect. *Child Abuse Review* **8**: 276–283.

Barlow, J., Stewart-Brown, S., Callaghan, H., Tucker, J., Brocklehurst, N., Davis, H. & Burns, C. (2003) Working in partnership: the development of a home visiting service for vulnerable families. *Child Abuse Review* **12(3)**: 172–189.

Barnard, K.E., Magyary, D., Sumner, G., Booth, C.L., Mitchell, S.K. & Spieker, S. (1988) Prevention of parenting alterations for women with low social support. *Psychiatry* **51**: 248–253.

Barker, P. (1990) Practical and ethical doubts about screening for child abuse. *Health Visitor* **63(1)**: 14–17.

Beckwith, L. (1988) Intervention with disadvantaged parents of sick preterm infants. *Psychiatry* **51**: 242–247.

Bell, S.M. & Ainsworth, M.D.S. (1972) Infant crying and maternal responsiveness. *Child Development* **43**: 117–190.

Bell, M. (2004) Child protection at the community level. *Child Abuse Review* **13(6)**: 363–367.

Belsky, J. (1993) Etiology of child maltreatment: a developmental, ecological analysis. *Psychological Bulletin* **114**: 413–434.

Belsky, J. (1984) The determinants of parenting: a process model. *Child Development* **55**: 83–96.

Belsky, J. & Isabella, R. (1988) Maternal, infant and social-contextual determinants of attachment security. In J. Belsky & T. Nezworski (eds), *Clinical Implications of Attachment* (pp. 41–93). Hillsdale, NJ, Lawrence Erlbaum Associates.

Benoit, D. & Parker, K.C.H. (1994) Stability and transmission of attachment across three generations. *Child Development* **65**: 1444–1456.

Benoit, D., Parker, K.C.H. & Zeanah, C.H. (1997) Mother's representations of their infants assessed prenatally: stability and association with infants' attachment classifications. *Journal of Child Psychology & Psychiatry* **38**: 307–313.

Bion, W.R. (1967) *Second Thoughts*. London, Karnac.

Bonnet, C. (1993) Adoption at birth: prevention against abandonment or neonaticide. *Child Abuse & Neglect* **17**: 501–513.

Bowlby, J. (1969) *Attachment and Loss: Vol. 1. Attachment*. New York, Basic Books.

Bowlby, J. (1973) *Attachment and Loss: Vol. 2. Separation: Anxiety and Anger*. New York, Basic Books.

Bowlby, J. (1980) *Attachment and Loss: Vol. 3. Loss: Sadness and Depression*. New York, Basic Books.

Bowlby, J. (1988) *A Secure Base: Clinical Applications of Attachment Theory*. London, Routledge.

Bretherton, I. & Waters, E. (eds). (1985) Growing points of attachment theory and research. *Monographs of the Society for Research in Child Development* (Serial no. 209), 50.

Briere, J. (1992) *Child Abuse Trauma: Theory and Treatment of Lasting Effects*. Newbury Park, CA, Sage Publications.

Brisby, T., Baker, S. & Hedderwick, T. (1997) *Under the Influence: Coping with Parents who Drink Too Much*. London, Alcohol Concern.

Brocklehurst, N., Barlow, J., Kirkpatrick, S., Davis, H. & Stewart-Brown, S. (2004) The contribution of health visitors to supporting vulnerable children and their families at home. *Community Practitioner* **77(5)**: 175–180.

Bronfenbrenner, U. (1979) *The Ecology of Human Development*. Cambridge MA, Harvard University Press.

Brown, J., Cohen, P., Johnson, J.G. & Salzinger, S. (1998) A longitudinal analysis of risk factors for child maltreatment: findings of a 17-year prospective study of officially recorded and self-reported child abuse and neglect. *Child Abuse and Neglect* **22**: 1065–1078.

Browne, K.D. (1994) Child sexual abuse. In J. Archer (ed.), *Male Violence* (pp. 210–230). London, Routledge.

Browne, K.D. (1995a) Alleviating spouse relationship difficulties. *Counselling Psychology Quarterly* **8(2)**: 109–122.

Browne, K.D. (1995b) Preventing child maltreatment through community nursing. *Journal of Advanced Nursing* **21**: 57–63.

Browne, K.D. (1995c) Predicting maltreatment. In P. Reder & C. Lucey (eds), *Assessment of Parenting* (pp. 118–135). London, Routledge.

Browne, K.D., Dixon, L. & Hamilton-Giachritsis, C.E. (in submission). An evaluation of an English home visiting programme in relation to the identification of families at risk of child maltreatment. *Child Abuse and Neglect*.

Browne, K.D., Falshaw, L. & Dixon, L. (2002) Treating domestic violent offenders. In K. Browne, H. Hanks, P. Stratton & C. Hamilton (eds), *Early Prediction and Prevention of Child Abuse: A Handbook* (pp. 317–336). Chichester, John Wiley & Sons, Ltd.

Browne, K.D. & Hamilton, C.E. (1999) Police recognition of the links between spouse abuse and child abuse. *Child Maltreatment* **4(2)**: 136–147.

Browne, K.D. and Hamilton, C.E. (2003). Prevention: Current and future trends. In M.J. Jannan and Y.H. Carter (eds), *Protecting Children from Abuse and Neglect in Primary Care*. Oxford, OUP.

Browne, K.D., Hamilton, C.E., Hegarty, J. & Blissett, J. (2000) Identifying need and protecting children through community nursing home visits. *Representing Children* **13(2)**: 111–123.

Browne, K.D., Hamilton-Giachritsis, C.E., Johnson, R., Agathonos-Georgopoulou, H., Anaut, M., Herczog, M., Keller-Hamela, M., Klimakova, A., Leth, I., Ostergren, M., Stan, V. & Zeytinoglu, S. (2005) *Mapping the Number and Characteristics of Children under Three in Institutions across Europe at Risk of Harm*. Birmingham, England: Birmingham University Centre for Forensic and Family Psychology/European Commission/World Health Organisation.

Browne, K., Hanks, H., Stratton, P. & Hamilton, C. (2002) *Early Prediction and Prevention of Child Abuse: A Handbook* (pp. 317–336). Chichester, John Wiley & Sons, Ltd.

Browne, K.D. & Herbert, M. (1997) *Preventing Family Violence*. Chichester, John Wiley & Sons, Ltd.

Browne, K.D. & Lynch, M. (1995) The nature and extent of child homicide and fatal abuse. *Child Abuse Review* **4(5)**: 309–316.

Browne, K.D. & Saqi, S. (1987) Parent-child interaction in abusing families: its possible causes and consequences. In P. Maher (ed.), *Child Abuse: the Educational Perspective* (pp. 77–103). Oxford, Blackwell.

Browne, K.D. & Saqi, S. (1988a) Approaches to screening for child abuse and neglect. In K. Browne, C. Davies & P. Stratton (eds), *Early Prediction and Prevention of Child Abuse* (pp. 57–88). Chichester, John Wiley & Sons, Ltd.

Browne, K.D. & Saqi, S. (1988b) Mother-infant interactions and attachment in physically abusing families. *Journal of Reproductive and Infant Psychology* **6**: 163–282.

Brunner, J.S., Goodnow, J.J. & Austin, G.A. (1956) *A Study of Thinking*. New York, John Wiley & Sons, Inc.

Buchanan, A. (1996) *Cycles of Child Maltreatment: Facts, Fallacies and Interventions*. Chichester, John Wiley & Sons, Ltd.

Carlson, V., Cicchetti, D., Barnett, D. & Braunwald, K. (1989) Disorganised/disoriented attachment relationships in maltreated infants. *Developmental Psychology* **25**: 525–531.

Cassidy, J. & Shaver, P.R. (1999) *Handbook of Attachment: Theory, Research and Clinical Applications*. New York, Guilford Press.

Clarke, A.M. & Clarke, A.D.B. (1976) *Early Experience: Myth and Evidence*. London, Open Books.

Cleaver, H., Unell, I. & Aldgate, J. (1999) *Children's Needs – Parenting Capacity: the Impact of Parental Mental Illness, Problem Alcohol and Drug Abuse, and Domestic Violence on Children's Development.* London, The Stationery Office.

Combes, G. & Schonveld, A. (1992) *Life Will Never Be the Same Again.* London, Health Education Authority.

Cooper, P.J., Campbell, E.A., Day, A., Kennerley, H. & Bond, A. (1988) Non-psychiatric disorder after childbirth: a prospective study of prevalence, incidence, course and nature. *British Journal of Psychiatry* **152**: 799–806.

Cowan, P. & Cowan, C.P. (2001) A couple perspective on the transmission of attachment patterns. In C. Clulow (ed.), *Adult Attachment and Psychotherapy: The Secure Base in Practice and Research* (pp. 62–82). East Sussex, Brunner-Routledge.

Cox, J.L., Holden, J.M. & Sagovsky, R. (1987) Detection of postnatal depression. Development of the 10-item Edinburgh Postnatal Depression Scale. *B.J.Psych.* **150**: 782–786.

Crittenden, P. (2002) If I knew then what I know now: integrity and fragmentation in the treatment of child abuse and neglect. In K. Browne, H. Hanks, P. Stratton & C. Hamilton (eds), *Early Prediction and Prevention of Child Abuse: A Handbook* (pp. 111–126). Chichester, John Wiley & Sons, Ltd.

Crouch, J.L., Milner, J.S. & Thomsen, C. (2001) Childhood physical abuse, early social support and risk for maltreatment: current social support as a mediator of risk for child physical abuse. *Child Abuse and Neglect* **25**: 93–107.

D'Ath, E. & Pugh, G. (1986) *Working with Parents: A Training Resource Pack.* London, National Children's Bureau.

Davis, H., Day, C. & Bidmead, C. (2002) *Working in Partnership with Parents: the Parent Advisor Model.* London, The Psychological Corporation.

Dawson, G., Hessl, D. & Freyer, K. (1994) Social influences on early developing biological and behavioural systems related to risk for affective disorder. *Development and Psychopathology* **6**: 759–779.

Department for Education and Employment (1999) *Sure Start.* London, DFEE Publications.

Department for Education and Skills (2004a) *Every Child Matters – The Next Step.* London, The Stationery Office.

Department for Education and Skills (2004b) *Every Child Matters – Change for Children in Social Care.* London, The Stationery Office.

Department for Education and Skills (2004c) *Every Child Matters – Change for Children in Schools.* London, The Stationery Office.

Department for Education and Skills (2004d) *Every Child Matters – Change for Children in the Criminal Justice System.* London, The Stationery Office.

Department of Health, Education and Skills (2004e). The National Service Framework for children, young people and maternity services: core standards. *Every Child Matters.* London, HMSO.

Department for Education and Skills & Department of Health (2004) *Every Child Matters – Change for Children in Health Services.* London, The Stationery Office.

Department for Education and Skills (2005). *Children and Young People on Child Protection Registers Year Ending 31st March 2004, England (Personal Social Services and Local Authority Statistics).* London, Government Statistical Service.

Department of Health (1995) *Child Protection: Messages from Research.* London, HMSO.

Department of Health (1996) *Child Health in the Community: A Guide to Good Practice.* London, National Health Service Executive.

Department of Health (1999) *Saving Lives: Our Healthier Nation.* London, The Stationery Office.

Department of Health (2004) *National Service Framework for Children, Young People and Maternity Services*. London, The Stationery Office.

Department of Health (2005a) *Safeguarding Children: A Summary of the Joint Chief Inspectors Report on Arrangements to Safeguard Children*. London, The Stationery Office.

Department of Health (2005b) *Children and Young People on Child Protection Registers Year Ending 31st March 2004, England (Personal Social Services and Local Authority Statistics)*. London, Government Statistical Service.

Department of Health, British Medical Association, Conference of Medical Royal Colleges (1994) *Child Protection: Medical Responsibilities (Addendum to Working Together Under the Children Act 1989)*. London, Department of Health.

Department of Health, Department of Education and Employment, and the Home Office (1999) *Working to Safeguard Children*. London, The Stationery Office.

Department of Health, Department of Education and Employment, and the Home Office (2000) *Framework for the Assessment of Children in Need and their Families*. London, The Stationery Office.

Department of Health, Department of Education and Employment, and the Home Office (2003) *Keeping Children Safe*. London, The Stationery Office.

Department of Health & Quinton, D. (2004) *Supporting Parents: Messages from Research*. London, Jessica Kingsley.

De Wolff, M.S. & van Ijzendoorn, M.H. (1997) Sensitivity and attachment: a meta analysis on parental antecedents of infant attachment. *Child Development* **68**: 571–591.

Dixon, L., Browne, K.D. & Hamilton-Giachritsis, C.E. (2005) Risk factors of parents abused as children: a mediational analysis of the intergenerational continuity of child maltreatment (Part I). *Journal of Child Psychology and Psychiatry* **46(1)**: 47–57.

Dixon, L., Hamilton-Giachritsis, C.E. & Browne, K.D. (2005) Behavioural measures of parents abused as children: a mediational analysis of the intergenerational continuity of child maltreatment (Part II). *Journal of Child Psychology and Psychiatry* **46(1)**: 58–68.

Downey, G. & Coyne, J.C. (1990) Children of depressed parents: an integrative review. *Psychological Bulletin* **108**: 50–76.

Drummond, D.C. & Fitzpatrick,G. (2000) Children of substance-misusing parents. In P. Reder, M. McClure & A. Jolley (eds), *Family Matters: Interfaces between Child and Adult Mental Health* (pp. 135–149). London, Routledge.

Dunn, J. (1977) *Distress and Comfort*. London, Fontana/Open Books.

Dunn, J. (1993) *Young Children's Close Relationships: Beyond Attachment*. Newbury Park, Sage.

Dunn, J. & Kendrick, C. (1982) *Siblings: Love, Envy and Understanding*. Cambridge, Mass., Harvard University Press.

Durfee, M. & Tilton-Durfee, D. (1995) Multi-agency child death review teams: experiences in the United States. *Child Abuse Review* **4**: 377–381.

Egan, G. (1990) *The Skilled Helper: A Systematic Approach to Effective Helping*. Pacific Grove, CA, Brookes/Cole.

Egeland, B., Bosquet, M. & Chung, A.L. (2002) Continuities and discontinuities in the intergenerational transmission of child maltreatment: implications for breaking the cycle of abuse. In K. Browne, H. Hanks, P. Stratton & C. Hamilton (eds), *Early Prediction and Prevention of Child Abuse: A Handbook* (pp. 217–232). Chichester, John Wiley & Sons, Ltd.

Elder, G., Caspi, A. & Downey, G. (1986) Problem behaviour and family relationships: life course and intergenerational themes. In A. Sorensen, F. Weinart & L. Sherrod (eds), *Human Development: Interdisciplinary Perspectives* (pp. 293–340). Hillsdale, NJ, Erlbaum.

Elkan, R., Kendrick, D., Hewitt, M., Robinson, J.J.A., Tolley, K., Blair, M. et al. (2000) The effectiveness of domiciliary health visiting: A systematic review of international studies and a selective review of the British literature. *Health Technology Assessment,* **4(13)**.

Emde R. (1989) The infants relationship experience: developmental and affective aspects. In A. Samarott and R. Emde (eds), *Relationship Disturbances in Early Childhood.* New York, Basic Books.

Etchegoyen, A. (2000) Perinatal mental health. In P. Reder, M. McClure & A. Jolley (eds), *Family Matters: Interfaces Between Child and Adult Mental Health* (pp. 257–270). London, Routledge.

Falkov, A. (1996) *Study of Working Together 'Part 8' Reports. Fatal Child Abuse and Parental Psychiatric Disorder: An Analysis of 100 Area Child Protection Committee Case Reviews Conducted Under the Terms of Part 8 of Working Together Under the Children Act 1989.* London, Department of Health.

Fantuzzo, J., Boruch, R., Beriama, A., Atkins, M. & Marcus, S. (1997) Domestic violence and children: prevalence and risk in five major US cities. *Journal of the American Academy of Child and Adolescent Psychiatry* **36**: 116–122.

Feinstein, L. (1998) *Pre-school Education Inequality?* London, Centre for Economic Performance, London School of Economics.

Fellow-Smith, L. (2000) Impact of parental anxiety disorder on children. In P. Reder, M. McClure & A. Jolley (eds), *Family Matters: Interfaces between Child and Adult Mental Health.* London, Routledge.

Fergusson, D.M. & Harwood, L.J. (1998) Exposure to interparental violence in childhood and psychosocial adjustment in young adulthood. *Child Abuse & Neglect* **22**: 339–357.

Finkelhor, D. (1980) Risk factors in the sexual victimization of children. *Child Abuse and Neglect* **4**: 265–273.

Finkelhor, D., Hotaling, G., Lewis, I.A. & Smith, C. (1990) Sexual abuse in a national survey of adult men and women: prevalence, characteristics and risk factors. *Child Abuse and Neglect* **14**: 19–28.

Fonagy, P. (1998) Prevention, the appropriate target of infant psychotherapy. *Infant Mental Health Journal* **19**: 124–150.

Fonagy, P., Steele, H. & Steele, M. (1991) Maternal representations of attachment during pregnancy predict the organisation of infant-mother attachment at one year of age. *Child Development* **62**: 891–905.

Fortin, A. & Chamberland, C. (1995) Preventing the psychological maltreatment of children. *Journal of Interpersonal Violence* **10**: 275–295.

Fraiberg, S. (1980) *Clinical Studies in Infant Mental Health.* New York, Basic Books.

Fraiberg, S., Adelson, E. & Shapiro, V. (1975) Ghosts in the nursery: A psychoanalytic approach to the problems of impaired infant-mother relationships. *Journal of the American Academy of Child Psychiatry* **14**: 387–421.

Frodi, A.M. & Lamb, M.E. (1980) Child abusers' responses to infants' smiles and cries. *Child Development* **51**: 238–241.

Gelfand, D.M. & Teti, D.M. (1990) The effects of maternal depression on children. *Clinical Psychology Review* **10**: 329–353.

Gil, D. (1970) *Violence Against Children.* Cambridge, MA, Harvard University Press.

Gilardi, J. (1991) Child Protection in a South London district. *Health Visitor* **64(7)**: 225–227.

Giles-Sims, A. & Finkelhor, D. (1984) Child abuse in step-families. *Family Relations* **33(3)**: 427–433.

Glaser, D. (2000) Child abuse and neglect and the brain – a review. *Journal of Child Psychology and Psychiatry* **41**: 97–117.

Glaser, D. (2002) Emotional abuse and neglect (psychological maltreatment): a conceptual framework. *Child Abuse & Neglect* **26(6/7)**: 697–714.

Glaser, D. & Prior, V. (1997) Is the term child protection applicable to emotional abuse? *Child Abuse Review* **6**: 315–329.

Glaser, D. & Prior, V. (2002) Predicting emotional abuse and neglect. In K.D. Browne, H. Hanks, P. Stratton & C. Hamilton (eds), *Early Prediction and Prevention of Child Abuse: a Handbook* (pp. 57–70). Chichester, John Wiley & Sons, Ltd.

Goldson, E. (1998) Children with disabilities and child maltreatment. *Child Abuse and Neglect* **22**: 663–667.

Greenland, C. (1987) *Preventing CAN deaths: An International Study of Deaths Due to Child Abuse and Neglect.* London, Tavistock.

Grietens, H., Geeraert, L. & Hellinckx, W. (2004) A scale for home visiting nurses to identify risks of physical abuse and neglect among mothers with newborn infants. *Child Abuse and Neglect* **28**: 321–337.

Gullotta, T.P., Hampton, R.L. & Jenkins, P. (1996) *Preventing Violence in America.* London, Sage.

Guterman, N.B. (1997) Early prevention of physical child abuse and neglect: Existing evidence and future directions. *Child Maltreatment* **2**: 12–34.

Guterman, N.B. (1999) Enrollment strategies in early home visitation to prevent physical child abuse and neglect and the 'universal versus targeted' debate: A meta-analysis of population-based and screening-based programs. *Child Abuse and Neglect* **23(9)**: 863–890.

Grych, J.H. & Fincham, D. (1990) Marital conflict and children's adjustment: A cognitive contextual framework. *Psychological Bulletin* **108**: 267–290.

Hahn, R.A., Bilukha, O.O., Crosby, A., Fullilove, M.T., Liberman, A., Moscicki, E.K. et al. (2003) First reports evaluating the effectiveness of strategies for preventing violence: early childhood home visitation. Findings from the Task Force on Community Preventive Services. *Morbidity & Mortality Weekly Report. Recommendations & Reports* **52**: 1–9.

Hall, D. (2003) *Health for All Children* (4th edn). Oxford, Oxford University Press.

Hamilton, C.E. & Browne, K.D. (1999) Recurrent maltreatment during childhood: a survey of referrals to police child protection units in England. *Child Maltreatment* **4(4)**: 275–286.

Hamilton, C.E. & Browne, K.D. (2002) Predicting physical maltreatment. In K.D. Browne, H. Hanks, P. Stratton & C. Hamilton (eds), *Early Prediction and Prevention of Child Abuse: a Handbook* (pp. 41–56). Chichester, John Wiley & Sons, Ltd.

Hampton, R.L. (1999) *Family Violence: Prevention and Treatment.* London, Sage.

Hampton, R.L., Senatore, V. & Gullotta, T.P. (1998) *Substance Abuse, Family Violence and Child Welfare: Bridging Perspectives.* London, Sage.

Harker, L. & Kendall, L. (2003) *An Equal Start: Improving Support During Pregnancy and the First 12 Months.* London, IPPR.

Hart, B. & Risley, T.R. (1995) *Meaningful Differences in the Everyday Experiences of Young American Children.* Baltimore, Paul H. Brookes Publishing.

Hay, D., Pawlbry, S., Sharp, D., Asten, P., Mills, A. & Kumar, R. (2001) Intellectual problems shown by 11-year-old children whose mothers had postnatal depression. *Journal of Child Psychology & Psychiatry* **42**: 871–889.

Hegarty, J. (2000a) *The CARE Programme (Child Assessment Rating and Evaluation) Training Pack.* Southend Community Care Services (NHS) Trust. Southend on Sea, Essex.

Hegarty, J. (2000b) *The CARE Programme (Child Assessment Rating and Evaluation). Assessment Procedures Manual for Health Visitors.* Southend Community Care Services (NHS) Trust. Southend on Sea, Essex.

Helton, A. (1986) The pregnant battered female. *Response to Victimization of Women and Children* **1**: 22–23.

Hendry, E. (1997) Engaging General Practitioners in Child Protection Training. *Child Abuse Review* **6(1)**: 60–64.

Henricson, C. & Bainham, A. (2005) *The Child and Family Policy Divide: Tensions, Convergence and Rights.* York, Joseph Rowntree Foundation.

Herbert, M. (1991) *Child Care and the Family.* Windsor, NFER Nelson.

Home Office (1998) *Supporting Families: A Consultation Document.* London, The Stationery Office Group.

Home Office (2003) Reducing Homicide: a review of possibilities. On line report by F. Brockman & M. Maguire, January, www.homeoffice.gov.uk.

Hoskote, A.U., Martin, K., Hormbery, P. & Burns, E. (2003) Fractures in infants: one in four is non-accidental. *Child Abuse Review* **12(6)**: 384–391.

Hyman, C., Parr, R. & Browne, K.D. (1979) An observation study of mother-infant interaction in abusing families. *Child Abuse and Neglect* **3**: 241–246.

Ijzendoorn, M.H., Juffer, F. & Duyvesteyn, M.G.C. (1995) Breaking the intergenerational cycle of insecure attachment: a review of the effect of attachment-based interventions on maternal sensitivity and infant security. *Journal of Child Psychology & Psychiatry* **36**: 225–248.

Iwaniec, D. (1995) *The Emotionally Abused and Neglected Child.* Chichester, John Wiley & Sons, Ltd.

Iwaniec, D. (2004) *Failure to Thrive.* Chichester, John Wiley & Sons, Ltd.

Iwaniec, D., Herbert, M. & Sluckin, A. (2002) Helping emotionally abused and neglected children and abusive carers. In K.D. Browne, H. Hanks, P. Stratton & C. Hamilton (eds), *Early Prediction and Prevention of Child Abuse: A Handbook* (pp. 249–266). Chichester, John Wiley & Sons, Ltd.

Jacobsen, S.W. & Frye, K.F. (1991) Effect of maternal social support on attachment: experimental evidence. *Child Development* **62**: 572–582.

Jason, J., Williams, S., Burton, A. & Rochat, R. (1982) Epidemiological differences between sexual and physical child abuse. *Journal of the American Medical Association* **247**: 3344–3348.

Johnston, J. & Campbell, L. (1988) *Impasses of Divorce: Dynamics and Resolution of Family Conflict.* New York, The Free Press.

Juffer, F., Bakermans-Kranenburg, M.J. & van Ijzendoorn, M.H. (2005) The importance of parenting in the development of disorganised attachment: evidence from a preventative intervention study in adoptive families. *Journal of Child Psychology and Psychiatry* **46(3)**: 263–274.

Kaler, S. & Freeman, B. (1994) Analysis of environmental deprivation: cognitive and social development in Romanian orphans. *Journal of Child Psychology & Psychiatry* **35**: 769–781.

Kandal, E.R., Schwartz, J.H. & Jessell, T.M. (1991) *Principles of Neural Science,* 3rd edn. London, Prentice-Hall.

Kaufman, J. & Zigler, E. (1989) The intergenerational transmission of child abuse. In D. Cicchetti & V. Carlson (eds), *Child Maltreatment: Theory and Research on the Causes and Consequences of Child Abuse and Neglect* (pp. 129–150). New York, Cambridge University Press.

Kitzman, H., Olds, D., Henderson, Jr, C.R., Hanks, C., Cole, R., Tatelbaum, R., McConnochie, K.M., Sidora, K., Luckey, D.W., Shaver, D., Engelhardt, K., James, D.

& Barnard, K. (1997) Effect of prenatal and infancy home visitation by nurses on pregnancy outcomes, childhood injuries, and repeated childbearing: a randomized controlled trial. *The Journal of the American Medical Association* **278**: 644–652.

Kitzman, H., Olds, D., Sidora, K., Henderson, Jr. C.R., Hanks, C., Cole, R., Luckey, D.W., Bondy, J., Cole, K. & Glazner, J. (2000) Enduring effects of nurse home visitation on maternal life course. *The Journal of the American Medical Association* **283**: 1983–1989.

Leventhal, J. (1988) Can child maltreatment be predicted during the perinatal period: Evidence from longitudinal cohort studies. *Journal of Reproductive and Infant Psychology* **6(3)**: 139–162.

Lieberman, A.F., Weston, D.R. & Pawl, J.H. (1991) Preventive intervention and outcome with anxiously attached dyads. *Child Development* **62**: 199–209.

Lynch, M. (1975) Ill-health and child abuse. *The Lancet* **2**: 317–319.

Lynch, M. & Roberts, J. (1977) Predicting child abuse. *Child Abuse and Neglect* **1**: 491–492.

Lyons-Ruth, K., Connell, D.B., Grunebaum, H.U. & Botein, S. (1990) Infants at social risks: maternal depression and family support services as mediators of infant development and security of attachment. *Child Development* **61**: 85–98.

Maccoby, E.E. (1980) *Social Development: Psychology Growth and the Parent-Child Relationship*. NY, Harcourt Brace Jovanovich.

MacMillan, H.I., Thomas, B.H., Jamieson, E., Walsh, C.A., Boyle, M.H., Shannon, H.S. & Gafni, A. (2005) Effectiveness of home visitation by public-health nurses in prevention of the recurrence of child physical abuse and neglect: a randomised controlled trial. *The Lancet*, **365**: 1786–1793.

MacMillan, H.L. & Canadian Task Force on Preventive Health Care (2000) Preventive health care, 2000 update: prevention of child maltreatment. *Canadian Medical Association Journal* **163**: 1451–1458.

Main, M. & Hesse, E. (1990) Parents' unresolved traumatic experiences are related to infant disorganised attachment status: Is frightened and/or frightening parent behaviour the linking mechanism? In M. Greenberg, D. Cicchetti & E. Cummings (eds), *Attachment in the Preschool Years* (pp. 161–182). Chicago, University of Chicago Press.

Main, M., Kaplan, N. & Cassidy, J. (1985) Security of attachment in infancy, childhood and adulthood: A move to the level of representation. In I. Bretherton & E. Waters (eds), Growing points in attachment theory and research, *SRCD Monographs* **49**: Serial no. 209.

Main, M. & Solomon, J. (1990) Procedures for identifying infants as disorganised/disoriented during the Ainsworth Strange Situation. In M. Greenberg, D. Cicchetti & E. Cummings (eds), *Attachment in the Preschool Years* (pp. 121–160). Chicago, University of Chicago Press.

Manassis, K., Bradley, S., Goldberg, S., Hood, J. & Swinson, R.P. (1995) Behavioural inhibition, attachment and anxiety in children of mothers with anxiety disorder. *Canadian Journal of Psychiatry* **40**: 87–92.

Marks, M.N. & Kumar, R. (1996) Infanticide in England & Wales. *Medicine, Science and the Law* **33**: 329–339.

Martins, C. & Gaffan, E.A. (2000) Effects of early maternal depression on patterns of infant-mother attachment: a meta-analytic investigation. *Journal of Child Psychology & Psychiatry* **41**: 737–746.

McAllister, F. (1995) *Marital Breakdown and the Health of the Nation*. London, One plus One.

McConkey, R. (1985) *Working with Parents: a Practical Guide for Teachers and Therapists.* London, Croom Helm.

McFarlane, J. (1991) Violence during teen pregnancy: health consequences for the mother and child. In B. Levy (ed.), *Dating Violence: Young Women in Danger* (pp. 136–141). Seattle, WA, Seal.

Mebert, C.J. (1989) Stability and change in parents' perceptions of infant temperament: early pregnancy to 13.5 months post partum. *Infant Behaviour and Development* **12**: 237–244.

Mebert, C.J. (1991) Dimensions of subjectivity in parents' rating of infant temperament. *Child Development* **62**: 352–361.

Mihalopoulos, C., Sanders, M.R., Turner, K.M.T., Murphy-Brennan, M. & Carter, R. (in submission). Does the Triple P – Positive Parenting Program provide value for money?

Milner, J.S. (1986) *The Child Abuse Potential Inventory Manual* (2nd edn). De Kalb, IL, Psytec.

Moffitt, T.E. & Caspi, A. (1998) Implications of violence between intimate partners for child psychologists and psychiatrists. *Journal of Child Psychology & Psychiatry* **39**: 137–144.

Morgan, S.R. (1987) *Abuse and Neglect of Handicapped Children.* New York, Plenum.

Morton, N. & Browne, K.D. (1998) Theory and observation of attachment and its relation to child maltreatment: a review. *Child Abuse and Neglect* **22(11)**: 1093–1104.

Murphy, S., Orkow, B. & Nicola, R.M. (1985) Prenatal prediction of child abuse and neglect: a prospective study. *Child Abuse & Neglect* **9**: 225–235.

Murphy, J.M., Jellinek, M., Quinn, D., Smith, G., Poitrast, F.G. & Goshko, M. (1991) Substance abuse and serious child mistreatment: prevalence, risk and outcome in a court sample. *Child Abuse & Neglect* **15**: 197–211.

Murray, L. (1992) The impact of postnatal depression on infant development. *Journal of Child Psychology & Psychiatry* **33**: 543–561.

Murray, L. & Cooper, P. (1996) The impact of postpartum depression on child development. *International Review of Psychiatry* **8**: 55–63.

Murray, C.J.L., Gakidou, E.E. & Frenk, J. (1999) Health inequalities and social group differences: what should we measure? *Bulletin of the World Health Organisation* **77(7)**: 537–542.

National Commission of Enquiry in the Prevention of Child Abuse (1996) *Childhood Matters, Vol 1 & 2.* London, NSPCC.

Nelson, H.B. & Martin, C.A. (1985) Increased child abuse in twins. *Child Abuse and Neglect* **9(4)**: 501–505.

Newberger, E.H., Barkan, S., Lieberman, E., McCormick, M., Yllo, K., Gary, L. & Schechter, S. (1992) Abuse of pregnant women and adverse birth outcome: current knowledge and implications for practice. *Journal of the American Medical Association* **267(17)**: 2370–2372.

Newcomb, M.D. & Locke, T.F. (2001) Intergenerational cycle of maltreatment: a popular concept obscured by methodological limitations. *Child Abuse and Neglect* **25**: 1219–1240.

Nursing and Midwifery Council (2002).

Oates, M. (1994) Postnatal mental illness: organisation and function of services. In J. Cox & J. Holden (eds), *Perinatal Psychiatry: Use and Misuse of the Edinburgh Postnatal Depression Scale.* London, Gaskell.

O'Connor, T.G., Bredenkamp, D., Rutter, M. & The English and Romanian Adoptees Study Team (1999) Attachment disturbances and disorders in children exposed to early severe deprivation. *Infant Mental Health Journal* **20(1)**: 10–29.

O'Connor, T.G., Rutter, M. & The English and Romanian Adoptees Study Team (2000) Attachment disorder behavior following early severe deprivation: Extension and longitudinal follow-up. *Journal of the American Academy of Child & Adolescent Psychiatry* **39(6)**: 703–712.

O'Connor, T.G. (2002) Annotation: the 'effects' of parenting reconsidered: findings, challenges and applications. *Journal of Child Psychology & Psychiatry* **43**: 555–572.

O'Connor, T.G., Marvin, R.S., Rutter, M., Olrick, J.T., Britner, P.A. & The English and Romanian Adoptees Study Team (2003) Child-parent attachment following early institutional deprivation. *Development & Psychopathology* **15**: 19–38.

Olds, D., Eckenrode, J., Henderson, C., Kitzman, H., Powers, J., Cole, R., Sidora, K., Morris, P., Pettitt, L. & Luckey, D. (1997) Long-term effects of home visitation on maternal life course and child abuse and neglect: Fifteen year follow up of a randomized trial. *Journal of the American Medical Association* **278(8)**: 637–643.

Olds, D.L., Henderson, C.R., Phelps, C., Kitzman, H. & Hanks, C. (1993) Effect of prenatal and infancy nurse home visitation on Government spending. *Medical Care* **31(2)**: 155–174.

Olds, D., Henderson, Jr, C.R., Cole, R., Eckenrode, J., Kitzman, H., Luckey, D.W., Pettitt, L., Sidora, K., Morris, P. & Powers, J. (1998) Long-term effects of nurse home visitation on children's criminal and anti-social behavior: 15 year follow-up of a randomized control trial. *The Journal of the American Medical Association* **280**: 1238–1244.

Oliver, J.E. (1983) Dead children from problem families in NE Wiltshire. *British Medical Journal* **286**: 115–117.

Parameswaran, S. (1997) Parenthood: assessment of 'good enough parenting'. In K.W. Divedi (ed.), *Enhancing Parenting Skills: A Guide for Professionals Working with Parents*. Chichester, John Wiley & Sons, Ltd.

Parr, M. (1998) A new approach to parent education. *British Journal of Midwifery* **6**: 160–165.

Patterson, G.R. (1982) *Coercive Family Process: A Social Learning Approach* (vol. 3) Eugene, OR, Castalia.

Patterson, G.R., DeBaryshe, B.D. & Ramsey, E. (1989) A developmental perspective on antisocial behaviour. *American Psychologist* **44(2)**: 329–335.

Pears, K.C. & Capaldi, D.M. (2001) Intergenerational transmission of abuse: a two-generational prospective study of an at-risk sample. *Child Abuse and Neglect* **25**: 1439–1462.

Peters, R. & Barlow, J. (2003) Systematic review of instruments designed to predict child maltreatment during the antenatal and postnatal periods. *Child Abuse Review* **12**: 416–439.

Piaget, J. (1954) *The Construction of Reality in the Child*. London, Routledge & Kegan Paul.

Prochaska, J.O. & DiClemente, C.C. (1984) *The Transtheoretical Approach: Crossing the Traditional Boundaries of Therapy*. Malabar, FL, Krieger.

Putallaz, M., Costanzo, P.R., Grimes, C.L. & Sherman, D.N. (1998) Intergenerational continuities and their influences on children's social development. *Social Development* **7**: 389–427.

Quinton, D. (1999) *Joining New Families: a Study of Adoption and Fostering in Middle Childhood*. Chichester, John Wiley & Sons, Ltd.

Quinton, D. & Rutter, M. (1984) Parents with children in care 1: current circumstances and parenting. *Journal of Child Psychology and Psychiatry*, **25**: 211–229.

Quinton, D., Rutter, M. & Liddle, C. (1984) Institutional rearing, parenting difficulties and marital support. *Psychological Medicine* **14**: 107–124.

Reder, P. & Duncan, S. (1999a) Conflictual relationships and risks of child abuse. *Journal of Child Centred Practice* **6**: 127–145.

Reder, P. & Duncan, S. (1999b) *Lost Innocents: a Follow Up Study of Fatal Child Abuse.* London, Routledge.

Reder, P. & Duncan, S. (2000) Child abuse and parental mental health. In P. Reder, M. McClure & A. Jolley (eds), *Family Matters: Interfaces Between Child and Adult Mental Health* (pp. 166–179). London, Routledge.

Reder, P. & Duncan, S. (2002) Predicting fatal child abuse and neglect. In K.D. Browne, H. Hanks, P. Stratton & C. Hamilton (eds), *Early Prediction and Prevention of Child Abuse: A Handbook* (pp. 23–40). Chichester, John Wiley & Sons, Ltd.

Reder. P. & Lucey, C. (1995) Significant issues in the assessment of parenting. In P. Reder & C. Lucey (eds), *Assessment of Parenting: Psychiatric and Psychological Contributions* (pp. 3–20). London, Routledge.

Richman, N., Stevenson, J. & Graham, P. (1982) *Pre-school to School: a Behavioural Study.* London, Academic Press.

Roberts, A.R. (1987) Psycho-social characteristics of batterers: a study of 234 men charged with domestic violence offences. *Journal of Family Violence* **2**: 81–94.

Robotham, A. & Sheldrake, D. (eds) (2000) *Health Visiting: Specialist and Higher Level Practice.* London, Churchill Livingstone.

Runtz, M.G. & Shallow, J.R. (1997) Social support and coping strategies as mediators of adult adjustment following childhood maltreatment. *Child Abuse and Neglect* **21**: 251–266.

Rutter, M. & the English and Romanian Adoptees (ERA) study team (1998) Developmental catch-up, and deficit, following adoption after severe global privation. *Journal of Child Psychology & Psychiatry* **39**: 465–477.

Sanders, M. (1999) The Triple-P positive parenting program: towards an empirically validated multilevel parenting and family support strategy for the prevention of behaviour and emotional problems in children. *Clinical Child and Family Psychology Review* **2**: 71–90.

Sanders, M. & Cann, W. (2002) Promoting positive parenting as an abuse prevention strategy. In K.D. Browne, H. Hanks, P. Stratton & C. Hamilton (eds), *Early Prediction and Prevention of Child Abuse: A Handbook* (pp. 145–164). Chichester, John Wiley & Sons, Ltd.

Sanders, T., Cobley, C., Coles, L. & Kemp, K. (2003) Factors affecting clinical referral of young children with a subdural haemorrhage to child protection agencies. *Child Abuse Review* **12(6)**: 358–373.

Schaffer, H.R. & Emerson, P.E. (1964) The development of social attachments in infancy. *Monographs of the Society for Research in Child Development*, 28.

Schaffer, H.R. (1977) *Mothering.* London, Fontana/Open Books Original.

Schaffer, H.R. (1990) *Making Decisions About Children: Psychological Questions and Answers.* Oxford, Blackwell.

Schore, A.N. (2001a) Effects of a secure attachment relationship on right brain development, affect regulation, and infant mental health. *Infant Mental Health Journal* **22(1–2)**: 7–66.

Schore, A.N. (2001b) The effects of early relational trauma on right brain development, affect regulation, and infant mental health. *Infant Mental Health Journal* **22(1–2)**: 209–269.

Schuengel, C., Bakermans-Kranenberg, M.J. & Van Ijzendoorn, M.H. (1999) Frightening maternal behaviour linking unresolved loss and disorganised attachment behaviour. *Journal of Consulting and Clinical Psychology* **67**: 54–63.

Simpson, C.M., Simpson, R.J., Power, K.G., Salter, A. & Williams, G.-J. (1994) GPs' and health visitors' participation in child protection case conferences. *Child Abuse Review* **3**(3): 211–230.

Simpson, J.A. & Rholes, W.S. (1998) *Attachment Theory and Close Relationships.* NY, Guilford Press.

Sluckin, W., Herbert, M. & Sluckin, A. (1983) *Maternal Bonding.* Oxford, Blackwell.

Solomon, J. & George, C. (1990) *Attachment Disorganization.* NY, Guilford Press.

Spinner, M.R. & Siegel, L. (1987) Non-organic failure to thrive. *Journal of Preventative Psychiatry* **3**(3): 279–297.

Starr, R.H. (1982) *Child Abuse and Prediction Policy Implications.* Cambridge, MA, Ballinger.

Stern, D.N. (1995) *The Motherhood Constellation: a Unified View of Parent-infant Psychotherapy.* New York, Basic Books, Inc.

Stratton, P. & Swaffer, R. (1988) Maternal causal beliefs for abused and handicapped children. *Journal of Reproductive and Infant Psychology* **6**: 201–216.

Straus, M. (1979) Family patterns and child abuse in a nationally representative sample. *International Journal of Child Abuse and Neglect* **3**: 213–225.

Straus, M. & Smith, C. (1990) Family patterns and child abuse. In M.A. Straus & R.J. Gelles (eds), *Physical Violence in American Families* (pp. 245–261). New Jersey, Transaction Publishers.

Swadi, H. (1994) Parenting capacity and substance misuse: an assessment scheme. *ACPP Review & Newsletter* **16**: 237–244.

Tajima, E.A. (2000) The relative importance of wife abuse as a risk factor for violence against children. *Child Abuse and Neglect* **24**: 1383–1398.

Truax, C.B. & Carkhuff, R.R. (1967) *Towards Effective Counselling and Psychotherapy.* Chicago, Ill., Aldine.

Van den Boom, D. (1991) Preventative intervention and the quality of mother-infant interaction and infant exploration in irritable infants. In W. Koops, H. Soppe, J.L. van der Linden, P.C.M. Molenar & J.J.F. Schroots (eds), *Developmental Psychology Behind the Dykes. An Outline of Developmental Psychological Research in the Netherlands* (pp. 249–269). Delft, Eburon.

Van der Eyken, W. (1982) *Home Start: a Four Year Evaluation.* Leicester, Home Start Consultancy.

Ward, M.J. & Carlson, E.A. (1995) Association among adult attachment representations, maternal sensitivity and infant mother attachment in a sample of adolescent mothers. *Child Development* **66**: 69–79.

Westman, A. (2000) The problem of parental personality. In P. Reder, M. McClure & A. Jolley (eds), *Family Matters: Interfaces Between Child and Adult Mental Health* (pp. 150–165). London, Routledge.

Whiten, A. (1977) Assessing the effects of perinatal events on the success of the mother-infant relationship. In H.R. Schaffer (ed.), *Studies in Mother-infant interaction* (pp. 403–426). London, Academic Press.

Wilczynski, A. (1997) *Child Homicide.* London, Greenwich Medical Media.

Wilkinson, R.G. (1994) *Unfair Shares: The Effects of Widening Income Differences on the Welfare of the Young.* London, Barnardo's Publications.

Wilson, M. & Daly, M. (1987) Risk of maltreatment of children living with step-parents. In R.J. Gelles & J.B. Lancaster (eds), *Child Abuse and Neglect: Biosocial Dimensions* (pp. 215–232). New York, Aldine De Gruyter.

Winnicot, D.W. (1960) *The Maturational Processes and Facilitative Environment.* London, Hogarth.

Winnicot, D.W. (1971) *Playing and Reality.* New York, Basic Books.

World Health Organisation (1998a) *First Meeting on Strategies for Child Protection. Padua, Italy 29–31 October 1998.* Copenhagen, WHO Regional Office for Europe.

World Health Organisation (1998b) *Essential Antenatal, Perinatal and Postpartum Care.* Copenhagen, WHO Regional Office for Europe.

World Health Organisation (1999) *Report of the Consultation on Child Abuse Prevention. WHO, Geneva, 29–31 March 1999.* Geneva, WHO.

World Health Organisation (2000) *Health in the 21st Century.* Geneva, WHO.

Zeanah, C.H. & Barton, M.L. (1989) Introduction: Internal representations and parent-infant relationships. *Infant Mental Health Journal* **10**: 135–141.

Zeanah, C.H., Kener, M.A., Anders, T.F. & Vieira-Baker, C. (1987) Adolescent mothers' perceptions of their infants before and after birth. *American Journal of Orthopsychiatry* **57**: 351–360.

Zeanah, C.H., Kener, M.A., Stewart, L. & Anders, T.A. (1985) Prenatal perception of infant personality: a preliminary investigation. *Journal of the American Academy of Child Psychiatry* **24**: 204–210.

Zeanah, C.H., Mammen, O.K. & Lieberman, A.F. (1993) Disorders of attachment. In C. Zeanah (ed.), *Handbook of Infant Mental Health.* New York, Guilford Press.

Zeanah, C.H., Benoit, D., Hirshberg, L., Barton, M.L. & Regan, C. (1994) Mothers' representations of their infants are concordant with infant attachment classifications. *Developmental Issues in Psychiatry and Psychology*, **1**: 1–14.

Zeanah, C.H. & Zeanah, P.D. (1989) Intergenerational transmission of maltreatment: insights from attachment theory and research. *Psychiatry* **52**: 177–196.

INDEX

Note: page numbers in *italics* refer to information contained in tables, page numbers in **bold** refer to diagrams.